"SIX PRACTICAL LESSONS
FOR AN EASIER CHILDBIRTH

is the only book on the Lamaze method of psycho-prophylactic childbirth which clearly and forcefully describes and teaches this method in detail. No one is better qualified to present these lessons than Elisabeth Bing, the outstanding teacher and pioneer of the method in the country. No one who reads her book—made vivid through brilliant photographs and exposition—can fail to grasp the method for himself."

—Ralph M. Crowley, M.D.
President, The American Academy of Psychoanalysis

"I am not surprised that this is an exceptional book, for its author is an exceptional woman. Her sincere and personal interest in making childbirth a fulfilling and radiant experience for every woman illuminates each page. I feel certain that these SIX LESSONS will become the bible for many young couples."

—Alan F. Guttmacher, M.D.
former President, Planned Parenthood Federation

THIRD REVISED EDITION

SIX PRACTICAL LESSONS FOR AN EASIER CHILDBIRTH

Elisabeth Bing

Photographs by Jill Strickman

Drawings by Howard S. Friedman and Vivien Cohen

BANTAM BOOKS

NEW YORK TORONTO LONDON SYDNEY AUCKLAND

This book is dedicated to all the parents
who have studied with me,
and to the memory of Marjorie Karmel.

SIX PRACTICAL LESSONS FOR AN EASIER CHILDBIRTH
A Bantam Book

PUBLISHING HISTORY

Grosset edition published March 1967
Revised Bantam edition, mass market / March 1977
Third revised edition, trade paperback / March 1994

The author and publisher thank Sue and Phil Stern for
their good-natured assistance in the preparation of this book.

Library of Congress Cataloging-in-Publication Data

Bing, Elisabeth D.
Six practical lessons for an easier childbirth/by Elisabeth D. Bing; photography by Jill Strickman;
drawings by Howard S. Friedman and Vivien Cohen.—3rd rev. ed.
p.   cm.
Includes bibliographical references.
ISBN 0-553-37369-2
1. Natural childbirth.   I. Title.
RG661.B56   1993
618.4'5—dc20   93-26507
CIP

Published simultaneously in the United States and Canada

PRINTED IN THE UNITED STATES OF AMERICA

20 19 18 17 16 15 14 13 12 11

CONTENTS

FOREWORD

Having begun obstetrics more than forty years ago, I have been privileged to witness a revolution in both its practice and its art. The revolution in practice was brought about through the wider use of prenatal care, transfusion and diagnostic X-ray, and by the introduction of improved anesthesia, better surgical techniques, chemotherapeutics and antibiotics. These improvements in practice produced a startling reduction in illness and death. In my early years we witnessed sixty-seven mothers die per ten thousand births; today less than three deaths occur in ten thousand births.

Change in the art has transformed childbirth from a grim, frightening experience into a happy, cheerful event. One may question why the change did not come sooner. Perhaps because the danger intrinsic in childbirth caused a fanatical concentration on safe deliverance. Then, when safety was accomplished, medicine relaxed its single focus and began to view the nonorganic, the psychological aspects of childbirth. Grantly Dick-Read deserves credit for first emphasizing the harmful effects of fear and ignorance, both of which he attempted to dispel. His introduction of natural childbirth was a pioneering step and his sympathetic, tender and somewhat fatherly attitude toward the pregnant woman even overflowed into doctrinaire obstetrics.

The contributions of Lamaze and his disciples have further enriched the welfare of the parturient. By way of parenthesis, I should like to say that I met Dr. Lamaze at his Metal Workers' Hospital in Paris. He was a very large man, almost elephantine in appearance, yet seemed gentle and kind. Despite the language barrier, he took much time and great pains to tell me about his work. It is not my purpose to explain the theory or practice of psychoprophylaxis, for Mrs. Bing in her Six Practical Lessons for an Easier Childbirth has done this incredibly well, far better than could I or anyone else. I am not surprised that this is an exceptional book, for its author is an exceptional woman. Her sincere and personal interest in making childbirth a fulfilling and radiant experience for every woman illuminates each page.

I feel certain that these Six Lessons will become a bible for many young couples. How lucky they are to find it together, for if both study and follow its directions, their joint entrance into parenthood will almost certainly be a triumphant success. Having been a co-worker of the author, I am especially pleased that her personality—rare spirituality and great humanity—comes through to the reader.

Alan F. Guttmacher, M.D.
died March 18, 1974
President, Planned Parenthood Federation
Formerly Chief of Obstetrics and Gynecology,
Mt. Sinai Hospital, New York City

PREFACE

The very nature of childbirth has been recast and remodelled over the past few decades. When we think about the changes that have occurred, perhaps we should first remark on the ubiquitous new obstetrical technology that came into being over this period. A host of technological advances have allowed doctors to peer into the womb, to monitor the well-being of the baby, to induce, to accelerate, and even to preempt labor. The extent to which these technological breakthroughs contributed to the increased safety we see today for mother and baby can be questioned; the extent to which they reshaped patterns of childbirth care cannot.

But the real change in childbirth over this period is only indirectly related to the new technology. Rather, it relates to a metamorphosis of mind-set among childbearing women, based on new information and new ways in which that information has become available to them. As maternity care became more and more the province of professionals, so did the dissemination of information. The accumulated experience shared among women, and passed from mother to daughter, no longer met women's needs in a society where birth had become so complex. Prenatal classes evolved as a substitute for this lost information and to respond to the new needs. They have been eminently successful.

The full impact of prenatal education cannot be assessed solely by its effect on the individual woman giving birth. Once a critical mass of mothers became aware that options could be available to them, they began to demand these options. Previously unheard-of practices, such as a father's presence for labor and birth, rooming in, and early discharge from hospital, have become commonplace today. Elisabeth Bing was in the vanguard of this new, revolutionary movement.

It is many years since I first read *Six Practical Lessons for an Easier Childbirth*, but I still recall how excited I and so many of my contemporaries were when the book appeared. It heralded and ushered in a new era. For the first time, the concepts and insights of psychoprophylaxis became available to women everywhere, regardless of whether or not they had access to formal prenatal classes. It brought childbirth education home, where perhaps it belongs. With its personal, conversational style, it was like having Elisabeth with you in your own living room.

Exploring this new edition of *Six Practical Lessons for an Easier Childbirth*, I felt once again the same excitement. Although Elisabeth has modernized the text to accommodate some of the new realities of childbirth in the 1990s, she has changed nothing just for the sake of change. I can still feel her presence, talking with me; other readers will find her talking, one-to-one, with them.

It is a rare book that deserves to be called a modern classic, but this is certainly among the few that merit this designation. Perhaps more than any other single book, it has changed the face of childbirth. Use it and treasure it.

Murray W. Enkin, MD, FRCS(C)
Professor Emeritus,
Departments of Obstetrics and Gynecology,
   Clinical Epidemiology and Biostatistics,
McMaster University

INTRODUCTION

I wrote the first edition of this book twenty-five years ago, and not in my wildest dreams would I have ever thought that years later, this little textbook could still be in demand and be of practical help to thousands of young parents. Of course, I personally was convinced of the value of the Lamaze method but had simply hoped that "Prepared Childbirth" was here to stay and that its obvious appeal to parents would establish it as a "way of birth," not as some kind of fad of the sixties.

The Lamaze method has now become an accepted modality of obstetric procedure in our time. Today, hardly anyone will argue that it is detrimental to a woman's health or could endanger the newborn. And just because it has proved to be of lasting value, it has also proved to be a living tool. Changes have occurred, changes in technique to some extent, changes in approach, changes in obstetric knowledge; it is as if the infant Lamaze method has grown into early adulthood and that its existence is now taken for granted.

This third revision has been brought up to date to reflect current obstetrical thinking, as well as my continuing day-to-day experience with prospective parents in my childbirth education classes. I would like not only to thank my very first editor at Bantam Books, Grace Bechtold, but also Toni Burbank and Maria Mack, for helping me to describe changes and to convince Bantam to publish this "growing child" so that it can be of as much help today to as many or more young parents as it has been for the last twenty-five years.

OUR CLASS
CONVENES

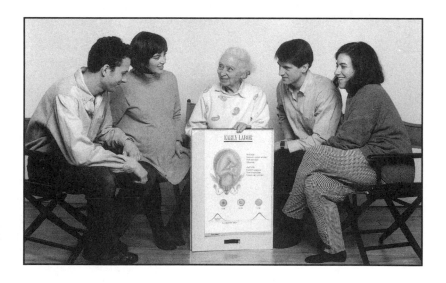

Women all over the world are preparing themselves for childbirth in a new and constructive way. They're learning about the changes that occur in the body during the nine months of gestation; they are doing exercises to prepare their bodies for giving birth; they are practicing new techniques of breathing and relaxation, which will help them ease pain and discomfort during labor and delivery.

This method of preparation is an intelligent woman's approach to the difficult emotional and physical task of giving birth. Many such women and their partners are now taking classes similar to those presented here, but this book will also allow prospective parents to prepare for childbirth at home without any formal curriculum.

To make things as simple and useful as possible, let us begin together as if you were all attending the classes I have given thousands of parents-to-be. If you follow the course closely, practicing the exercises and using the techniques prescribed, I

am sure you will have an active, happy and rewarding experience together.

AN INTRODUCTION TO THE LESSONS

You are one of a group of five young couples arriving at my
studio for your first lesson. The young women have various
occupations: One is a dancer, on leave from a Broadway show;
another is a lawyer; the third is a banker; and there are two
housewives, one of whom already has a little boy. The men's
professions are varied: a teacher, a book salesman, a stock-
broker, a mechanic, and a graduate student. All that these
people have in common is the fact that each of them will be the
parent of a new baby within the next two months.

We have found that the best time to start our course is
toward the end of the seventh or the beginning of the eighth
month, when a woman is psychologically ready to train herself
for labor and delivery. She is beginning to feel the weight of her
baby; she may have backaches; her abdominal muscles may feel
weak. At this point she is more likely to accept and welcome
the idea of training herself for the task ahead. If she had started
too early in her pregnancy, the will to work hard at her exercises would very likely have diminished as the months wore on.
Intensive training during the last phases of pregnancy not only
provides the best physical preparation, but keeps methods and
techniques fresh in the mind as actual labor and delivery arrive.

None of us in our class has met the others before, so there
is a certain feeling of nervous anticipation in the air. I
see that perhaps some of the men are a bit self-conscious—

understandably. Without further delay I face the class and begin.

I introduce myself and present the couples to each other.

"Now," I continue, "I would like to ask each of you why you are here tonight and what you expect from these classes. Would each of you, both husband and wife, tell me your reasons for enrolling?"

The women respond first:

"I want to know exactly what will happen to me and to my baby during labor and delivery."

"I would like to have as little medication as possible. My physician suggested that if I want to help during labor and delivery, if I want to be awake and participate in the birth of my child, then I should attend this course."

"My husband and I want to participate in the birth of our child. A friend of ours attended your classes and told us what wonderful preparation they are."

"I was totally unprepared for the birth of my first child. It was a dreadful experience. This time I want to know what's going on and help myself as well as I can."

And from the men:

"I want to help my wife prepare for childbirth and be with her during labor and delivery."

"My wife's first childbirth was a harrowing experience for both of us. This time I want her to be prepared to help the doctor during labor and have a more pleasant and positive experience. We've heard that this course can do just that."

"Our doctor has said that the exercises, information and respiratory techniques we can learn here are the best possible training and preparation for childbirth."

"Susan asked me to come along tonight. I really don't know what I am supposed to do here. If it were I who had to have the baby, I'd certainly ask the doctor to take care of me and put me to sleep for it. . . ."

"This is an experience we want to share together."

Now we are no longer strangers to each other. We are all here together for the same purpose: to learn about the fabulous engineering feat of giving birth; to gain confidence, a sense of joyous anticipation, a thorough knowledge of how to handle the emotional and physical difficulties—not passively, helpless and unconscious or pacing the hall outside, but as active participants.

WHAT IS THE "LAMAZE METHOD"?

Expectant mothers all over the world are preparing in exactly the same way for a conscious, healthy and happy experience. Our technique of preparation is called the Lamaze technique. I think you should all know a little about how this technique began and how it spread so rapidly throughout the world.

The late Grantly Dick-Read originated the idea that pain during labor was caused primarily by fear. He wrote in his famous book, *Childbirth Without Fear,* that pain in childbirth could be greatly reduced or even totally eliminated through understanding the process of labor and delivery and through learning to relax properly. Dick-Read felt childbirth is essentially a "normal and physiologic process," and that any pain felt is present because of poor conditioning, the influence of biblical stories, popular misconceptions, rumors and old wives' tales. Much of this concept has been generally accepted as valid, but we know now that all the education and "cultural conditioning" in the world cannot always provide a childbirth without any pain or discomfort whatsoever.

Dr. Dick-Read called his method "natural childbirth." Unfortunately, over the years the truth in this term has been almost totally obscured by layer upon layer of mysticism. It is thought to be a primitive childbirth, a childbirth completely without help or medication, a kind of endurance test. Dr. Dick-Read's pioneering work was—to a great extent—distorted, and the medical profession, as a result, has become wary of the term and concept of "natural childbirth."

This book presents a series of practical lessons in what we term the Lamaze method of childbirth. This method is *not* a technique of so-called "natural childbirth." On the contrary, it is a technique which is not at all natural, but acquired through concentrated effort and hard work on the part of the expectant mother and her husband. It is a method which provides an analgesic (or lessening of pain) achieved by physical means instead of by drugs or chemical means.

The technique originated in Russia, where it was first observed by the late Dr. Fernand Lamaze in 1951. Dr. Lamaze introduced the method to France and other European countries as well as China, Australia, Cuba and South America. In 1959 Marjorie Karmel published her book *Thank You, Dr. Lamaze* here in the United States. It was enormously influential in interesting American physicians and their patients in this new technique. I recommend that each of you read it if you have not already done so. A revised and updated edition was published in 1981 by Harper & Row.

In 1959 the American Society for Psychoprophylaxis in Obstetrics, Inc. (ASPO/Lamaze), was established. Numerous chapters and affiliates have been formed all over the United States. Now more and more American women and their husbands are preparing for an educated childbirth. American doctors are urging many of their expectant mothers to prepare with this method, and American hospitals have adapted their procedures to allow the active participation of husband and wife in labor and delivery.

What is the theory of the Lamaze method? What does the term psychoprophylaxis mean? It simply means a psychological and physical preparation for childbirth, but you will come to understand it more completely as we work through each lesson together.

HOW DO WE CONTROL PAIN?

Many interesting studies have been made of the nature of pain. We have discovered, for example, that no matter what part of the body provides the source of pain—your foot, knee, abdomen or head—all pain is registered in the cerebral cortex, a part of the brain. It has also been determined that it is not possible to measure the actual *degree* of pain, although its effects, such as changes in blood content, hormonal output, respiration, etc., can be registered.

Experiments have shown that the perception of pain depends on many things that may occur simultaneously with the pain itself. The fact is that we can usually concentrate only on one thing at a time. While we concentrate on one object or sensation, other feelings become peripheral. I'm sure all of you have experiences every day which demonstrate this fact. Let's think of a few examples.

We all know that it is possible to become so engrossed in reading a good book on a train, a subway, or even in a room full of noisy people, that any kind of potential distractions—conversation, whistles, clanging of doors—cannot interrupt our intense concentration. We often hardly notice what is happening around us. We notice the same phenomenon with something that is actually happening within us. Suppose, with a bad headache, you go to the movies and see a really fine film. You may not notice the headache at all while you are watching the picture, but when the film ends, it strikes you with renewed force. What has happened? Simply that your concentration on the film was strong enough to eliminate the perception of pain. When you ceased concentrating, the headache again became the center of your attention.

Another sure way to increase the perception of pain is to overanticipate it. All I have to do is sit down in my dentist's chair and I immediately feel apprehensive and tense. When the dentist asks me to open my mouth so he can look at my teeth I begin to feel pain.

I think most women approach childbirth the same way. They anticipate nothing but pain. "Surely it must hurt. Why are there so many different medications for childbirth if it is not excruciatingly painful?" they ask themselves. And by anticipating and concentrating entirely on the sensation of pain, they leave themselves wide open for real suffering.

No one knows how painful labor actually is. We agree with Dr. Dick-Read that much of the pain in childbirth comes of anxiety and fear, but we do not think that education and "deconditioning" can eliminate it all. We believe that understanding the process of labor and childbirth can alleviate any unnecessary apprehension, and with it *unnecessary* pain. We believe that certain easy exercises can also help prepare the body for a more comfortable labor and delivery. But after all this understanding, education and physical preparation, there is still an undeniable discomfort during childbirth. Our task now is to attack and deal with this residual pain.

Now, if pain in labor were as mild as a headache, I am sure the problem could be solved by installing television sets in every labor room and allowing each expectant mother to watch a fascinating program during delivery. As you can imagine, this technique does not work, but there is nothing wrong with the idea behind it. Our goal throughout these lessons—in addition to understanding what happens during childbirth and learning various exercises to prepare our bodies—will be to recondition ourselves and to create a new center of concentration, thereby causing the awareness of pain to become peripheral. We have found that this is possible not just by looking at an outside object, but by concentrating on a very special activity of our own.

This special activity consists of active and difficult techniques of breathing, which will demand a great amount of concentrated effort. We use different breathing techniques because our breathing is so closely connected with all our activities, whether physical or emotional. Our respiration always automatically synchronizes itself with our activity. When we are asleep, our breathing is very slow. Sitting still, our breathing is also quite slow, but faster than when we are sleeping. When we walk, run, or climb stairs, our breathing changes in rate and intensity. The same changes occur emotionally. Our breathing is slow if we are calm. It speeds up when we are excited or disturbed.

You will learn to change your breathing deliberately during

labor, adjusting it to the changing characteristics of the uterine contractions. This will demand an enormous concentrated effort on your part. Not a concentration on pain, but a concentration on your own activity in synchronizing your respiration to the signals that you receive from the uterus. This strenuous activity will create a new center of concentration in the brain, thereby causing the painful sensations during labor to become peripheral, to reduce their intensity. The breathing will not only serve you as a focal point. It will, at the same time, bring a good deal of oxygen to the baby who needs this additional oxygen in labor, as it is being squeezed and the oxygen supply is diminished while the uterus is contracting. Furthermore, the uterine muscle needs added amounts of oxygen in order to work efficiently. And at the same time, you will learn to relax your body in such a way that you will allow the uterus to work under optimum conditions.

These then are the basic principles of the Lamaze technique of childbirth: education, understanding, preliminary exercises and a technique of special breathing activity and relaxation during labor. I will give you these precision tools to work with. It will be up to you to take these tools and use them as your need demands.

HOW WELL DOES IT WORK?

We are often asked to give statistics about our method. Many physicians want to know whether birth injuries, prematurity, hemorrhaging, etc. can be reduced by using our method. Studies made in France and many other countries show that the psycho-prophylactic method does reduce these complications. But there is one important factor that cannot be measured statistically. That is: How does a rewarding experience in childbirth enhance a young couple's relationship with each other? How does the feeling of achievement, of having collaborated in the performance of a difficult job, such as giving birth, affect the husband and wife who have worked hard together toward this goal?

As I have already mentioned, the partner's role is crucial. He must help his wife while she is learning the respiratory techniques. He must see that she is properly relaxed during both practice and actual childbirth. He can help her concentrate on her breathing and signal the length of time between contractions. He must be constantly ready to provide both moral and physical support, not only by his own emotional and physical involvement, but also by the application of specific techniques that we will learn here in class. This can surely be the most joyous and satisfying experience a man and woman can have together.

We women do not give birth very often during our lives. In fact, in our country at this specific period of time, most babies that are born are born by choice and not by chance. This is a very new development, and I'm sure a sociologically and psychologically significant one. I would like to dream and think that a country whose citizens were all desired might make a wonderful future place for our children to live in. It would be a shame if this great event were to be a traumatic experience, one to be put out of our minds rather than happily remembered. I want to help you make the experience of childbirth a rewarding one which you can perform with dignity and joy, and which you and your husband can share together in happy collaboration.

But I also don't want to make amateur obstetricians out of you. I am sure you have all chosen your doctor or midwife carefully, and that you respect his or her judgment. But I want you to realize that giving birth is really a team effort. The team consists of you and your partner, myself as the teacher, and of course the nurses, midwives and your physician. We all have our roles to play.

This brings me to another important point I want to make before we begin our first lesson. I have often been asked the number of successes and failures among my students. I want you to realize that I do not accept the concept of failure in regard to the women I prepare for childbirth. Before we train in our method, we all start off at a point I call minus zero. Every one of you will achieve zero plus, and this will be *your* point of total success. There is no absolute goal, no threshold that all or any of us must reach. You certainly must not feel any kind of guilt or sense of failure if you require some medication, or if you experience discomfort or pain. This is a completely individual thing, depending on the physical nature of your body and its proportions, the size and shape of your baby, and many other factors.

If for any reason medical complications should arise, it is no longer up to you to handle them. Such problems are completely out of your hands, and any decisions of a medical nature lie with your physician or midwife. And let us keep in mind that in case mechanical difficulties do occur, your training and active cooperation can frequently help to avoid the use of instruments, or even the necessity of a cesarean section. Your conscious help and participation can provide invaluable assistance to your physician. You and your doctor will continue to function as a team.

And finally, I think that both of you should visit your doctor together for prenatal examinations. You as women are not having the baby alone. There are two of you creating a family. From the shared beginning through your pregnancy, you are involved together, learning not only to give birth, but how to parent.

LESSON 1

*How your body changes during pregnancy;
the importance of good posture;
the three stages of labor: contractions,
delivery of baby, expulsion of placenta.*

Let's begin this lesson by looking at some pictures (on the following pages) to help you understand the changes that occur in your body during pregnancy.

BODY CHANGES DURING PREGNANCY

Our first drawing represents the non-pregnant woman. Notice the shape of the uterus. Pay particular attention to the bottleneck opening, which is called the cervix. You can also see the close proximity of the uterus to the bladder, the intestines filling the abdomen, the stomach immediately under the diaphragm, and directly above that, the diaphragm and lungs.

The second drawing shows a pregnant woman, the fetus here about five months old. The uterus is really an extremely elastic, muscular bag. As the baby grows, the uterus expands, moving

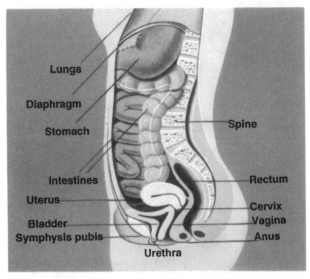

1. This illustration shows the position of the uterus in a non-pregnant woman and its relation to the other organs.

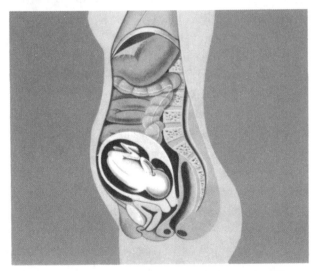

2. At five months the baby has entered the abdominal cavity, exerting some pressure against the diaphragm and lungs.

out of the pelvic cavity into the abdominal cavity, thereby pushing the intestines up and back.

In the third drawing, the fetus is in the ninth month. The uterus now fills the entire abdomen, while the intestines are pushed farther up against the stomach and diaphragm, compressing the lungs to a certain degree. This will explain why you are short of breath, why you may occasionally experience heartburn and why your stomach often feels uncomfortable after eating. You can also see how the pressure of the uterus against your bladder is causing all those frequent trips to the bathroom.

Take a closer look at the cervix in drawing number 3. You will observe a small plug at the bottleneck opening. This plug consists of mucus and tiny blood vessels. It prevents bacteria from entering the cervix and causing infection during pregnancy. This mucous plug is a safety device, and should be reassuring to you. Its presence allows activities such as intercourse, swimming, taking a bath. All these things are considered perfectly safe, unless, of course, your physician has given you specific instructions to avoid such activities during your pregnancy. Making love during pregnancy is generally considered safe. Perhaps the desire in the woman or in the man may vary in the three trimesters. Obviously you will have to be more inventive and find new positions for intercourse and pleasuring. But don't be afraid to make love. It's virtually impossible to hurt the baby.

As her self-image may suffer somewhat when a woman's figure changes in pregnancy, she may need a great deal of reassurance that she is still desirable. And I can't think of a more delightful way of being reassured than by being loved and making love.

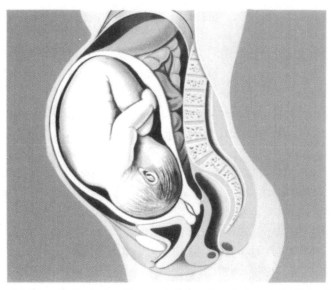

3. In ninth month the baby fills nearly the entire abdomen but nonethe-less internal organs continue to function well.

Look at the fourth drawing very carefully. You will notice that the cervix has become shorter, permitting your intestines and stomach more room. The pressure on the bladder has increased. Toward the end of your pregnancy the baby is likely to drop, settling into the pelvic cavity. It is also called lightening. But, I think these terms are both misnomers, as this is not a sudden drop, but gradual. At this point, you will notice that, although you can breathe more easily, there is increased pressure on your bladder and thighs.

Perhaps well-meaning people will tell you how "low" you carry, and overwhelm you with tales of what this might mean. Take no notice of their well-meant advice, but rather ask your doctor if you are in doubt about any symptom or discomfort. Your doctor will tell you now that the head of your baby has

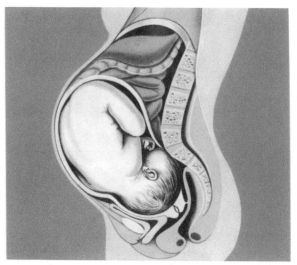

4. At the end of the ninth month the baby's head has become engaged, wedged now between pubic bone and sacrum.

become "engaged." What does this mean? It's really quite simple: the head has entered the pelvis, a cavity composed of the sacrum, the iliac bone, and the symphysis pubis. The engagement of the baby's head is an encouraging sign.

You now know that you are getting closer to labor. This may happen as long as three weeks before your due date, or it may happen only a few days before you go into labor. Occasionally the head will engage only when you are already in labor.

The fifth drawing shows the entire uterine bag. This bag is supported by ligaments, which act like columns supporting a building. There are two long ligaments, one on each side, and two short ones attached to the lower part of your spine. You may occasionally feel a sharp pain in your groin when you stretch suddenly, cough or sneeze. This picture shows you that

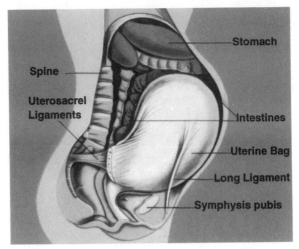

5. This shows the baby as it is contained in the uterine bag, which is supported by ligaments at the sides and the back.

such an occasional sudden pain is caused by stretching the long ligaments. The pain is of no consequence, and I hope you will be better able to put up with this occasional discomfort now that you realize what causes it.

THE IMPORTANCE OF GOOD POSTURE

The ligaments attached to your lower spine may cause backache during pregnancy. Backache in pregnancy is a frequent occurrence. Unfortunately we often increase the normal strain on our back by poor posture. It is so easy for us to take the line of least resistance when carrying a heavy baby. By letting the abdomen hang and leaning back slightly we weaken our abdominal muscles, simply by not using them. We may also strain the back muscles by overextending them. It is of the utmost importance that we learn to use our bodies correctly during pregnancy.

When standing we must always remember that the crown of our head is the highest part of the body. If you raise your head as indicated in the next pictures you find that the rest of your body aligns itself. There is no need to tuck in your bottom or your

The crown of your head is the highest part of your body.

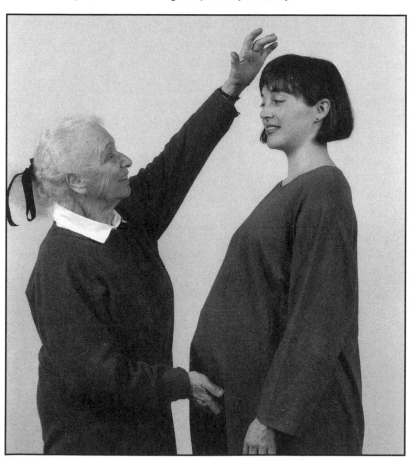

abdominal muscles. This will naturally occur if you thus raise your head.

You will find that good posture will enable you to walk more gracefully, putting far less strain on your abdominal and back muscles. And believe it or not, you will find that good posture will ease the pressure on your bladder. I suggest that your husband remind you now and then to "stretch up."

Good posture will also prevent fatigue. It is normal for you to tire more easily when you are pregnant, but don't let your tiredness accumulate. Rest during the day, if only for ten minutes at a time. Sit down, or better still, lie down with your legs raised. You will soon feel your energy coming back and be able to get through a long day with greater ease.

PELVIC FLOOR EXERCISE

Here is another exercise which will help you to strengthen the pelvic floor, make it more elastic, and make you more aware of your pelvic floor muscles, which you'll have to relax when you have to push your baby out. The exercise is called the "Kegel exercise," after the late Dr. Kegel, who described and used the exercise in the treatment of incontinence and poor pelvic muscle tone.

I will teach you now to exercise your pelvic floor or pubococcygeal muscle, which is the muscle band leading from near the pubic bone to near the coccyx. This muscle is shaped like a figure of eight, it surrounds your sphincters and passages, and its most important function is to support the bladder, the vagina and uterus, and the rectum.

Sit comfortably, legs slightly apart; lean forward a little.

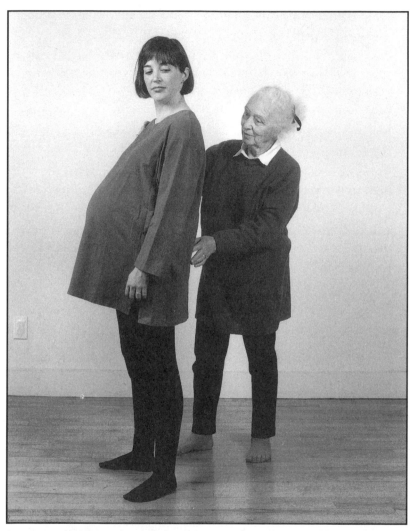

Sue demonstrates a very poor posture—one that will give her a backache and will weaken her abdominal muscles.

Now tighten your front passage as if to stop yourself from urinating. Then squeeze your vagina, and finally tighten your back passage as if you were preventing a bowel movement. Hold it—one—two—three—four—five—six—and release. Think "release" and you will find that you can relax even more. Always connect your body movements with your mind. If you think the movement, you will find that you can perform the exercise much more thoroughly.

Repeat this exercise at least 20 to 30 times a day. You can do it in a standing, sitting or lying position; while driving your car, in the subway or bus, at boring parties or during TV commercials. Nobody will ever notice you are doing it. My gynecologist gave me good advice: He said, "Each time you urinate, stop the flow, release, stop-release, etc." This will exercise your pelvic floor muscles, and it is easy to get into the habit of stopping and releasing the flow a number of times. I can easily repeat it 20 to 30 times in a day, though it depends a little on how much tea or coffee I have been drinking. However, you will soon notice that you are carrying your baby better, there will be less pressure on your thighs, and as a special bonus, you and your partner will find that love making is even more fun when you have the ability to contract and relax your vaginal muscles easily.

Exercising your pelvic floor muscles will improve the muscle tone and increase the elasticity of your perineum—the area between the anus and the vulva—so that it will stretch easily when your baby descends. Frequent use of these muscles will also make you conscious of their position and function, and will enable you to help the smooth expulsion of your baby through conscious neuromuscular control, just as the "concentration-relaxation" exercises, which you will learn later on, will help you develop relaxation and control over your arms, legs and facial muscles.

Practice this exercise diligently from now until you give birth. It is also one of the most important exercises to do shortly *after* you've given birth. Once you have delivered the baby and are back in your room (or even on the birthing bed or the delivery table) start contracting your pelvic floor. You will probably feel sore and numb in your pelvic area. The stitches from your episiotomy may feel irritated. You may be afraid to urinate or have a bowel movement. By using your Kegel exercises there and then, you can speed up the healing process of the episiotomy and begin a much more comfortable postpartum (after delivery) period.

I would like every woman to practice this pelvic floor exercise for the rest of her life in order to retain good muscle tone. This may prevent weakness or even a prolapse in later life.

Now let us look at the following pictures so that we may see the actual process of labor. In the illustration on page 28 you see a baby ready to be born. The mother is upright, with her back supported. You will recognize the spine, the anus, the vagina, the urinary opening or urethra, the uterus with its bottleneck cervix (which in this picture has lost its plug) and of course the baby, which is facing the mother's hip.

THE FIRST STAGE OF LABOR

Labor is divided into three stages. During the first stage, the uterus begins to contract involuntarily—that is, entirely on its own—thereby pulling on the cervix. The cervix becomes soft,

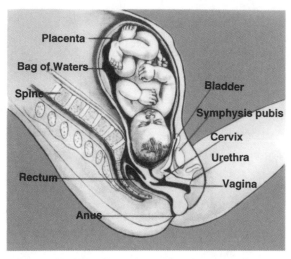

Placenta

Bag of Waters

Spine

Bladder

Symphysis pubis

Cervix

Urethra

Rectum

Vagina

Anus

1. **This baby is ready to be born: the mother is propped up at a 75° angle, her baby facing her right hip; the cervix is still thick and long; preliminary contractions have not yet occurred.**

thins out and flattens. This is called the *effacement* of the cervix. In the majority of women, the effacement starts toward the end of pregnancy, as early as two to three weeks before the birth of the baby. You may have already felt an occasional tightening in your abdomen. These tightenings are contractions of the uterus and are entirely painless. These preliminary contractions are called Braxton-Hicks contractions. They are named after an Englishman, Mr. Braxton-Hicks, who was the first to describe them in medical literature. Once labor proper begins, you will feel the uterine contractions more distinctly. These new, stronger contractions will cause the cervix to dilate.

The opening of the cervix can be compared to the neck of a very tight turtleneck sweater. Imagine yourself trying to put the sweater on: You pull it and stretch it until you have finally opened it far enough for you to push your head through. Thus

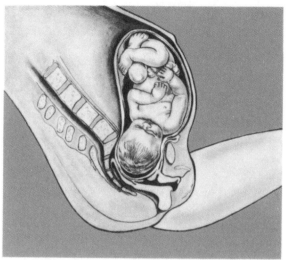

2. Here begins the first stage of labor: contractions have started; the baby has begun to move down and the cervix becomes shorter and flatter in the process called effacement.

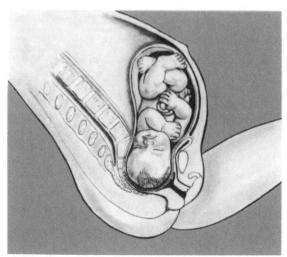

3. Baby rotates slightly as contractions during the first stage of labor continue. The cervix dilates; here it has opened about halfway, which is termed 2¹/₂ fingers or 5 centimeters.

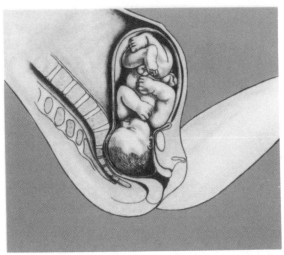

4. At the end of the first stage of labor, cervix is fully dilated (5 fingers or 10 centimeters); the baby's head is entering the stretched vagina and putting pressure upon the rectum.

the uterus has to pull on the cervix and stretch it with each contraction until it has opened to the widest diameter of the baby's head. Only then can you start to push your baby out. We say that the first stage of labor has ended when the cervix has opened fully to "5 fingers" or "10 centimeters."

I would like you to remember both these terms for the dilation of the cervix. Your doctor will examine you internally during labor and let you know how far along you are in precisely this language. He or she will say your cervix has opened up to "3 fingers" or "7 centimeters." I feel that communication between you and your physician is of the utmost importance before and during your labor. It is therefore essential for you to be acquainted with this terminology. Thus you can be fully aware of all the signposts on your road through labor to delivery. I will go into more detail on the first stage of labor on page 59.

THE SECOND STAGE OF LABOR

The door is now open. The second stage of labor is the expulsion of the baby. The uterus now works like a piston expelling the baby. Your lungs, diaphragm and strong abdominal muscles will provide the necessary power for this piston. You will see, in illustration 5, that the baby has rotated now and that the symphysis pubis acts as a pivotal point or fulcrum for the baby. The baby now faces the mother's spine and its head is at an angle. As the head gradually pushes through the vagina or birth canal the crown appears at the vulva or outlet of the vagina. At this point the doctor will talk of the "crowning" of the baby's head. The head now emerges, and you will

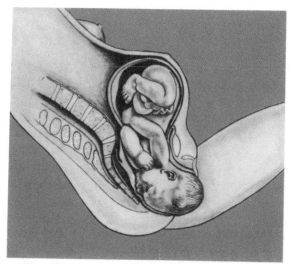

5. During the second stage of labor, the baby faces the mother's spine, flexing and extending its soft head to pivot around the pubic bone as it is pushed on through the birth canal.

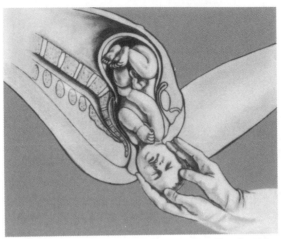

6. The head rotates once again on delivery to allow the shoulders and arms to emerge; the rest of the body slips out easily; expulsion is completed and the baby is born.

see from the next illustrations that it is being rotated once again (this time externally, often with the help of the doctor), to aid the expulsion of the shoulders. Once the shoulders have been delivered, the rest of the baby's body will slip out easily. The birth of the baby is the end of the second stage of labor.

A moment before you deliver the baby's head your doctor may make a small incision, called the "episiotomy," in the mouth of the vagina. This minor surgical procedure is performed to avoid possible tearing of your tissue as the baby's head is delivered. Your physician will decide whether or not an episiotomy is necessary. It is quite commonly done in America, and the incision can be done vertically or laterally, depending on your physician's decision at the time. A small, neat incision can be easily repaired, and heals quickly, whereas a tear with a ragged edge may create difficulties. The incision is frequently done with a local anesthetic.

It is important for you to realize that an episiotomy does not in any way interfere with your desire and ability to use the Lamaze method of childbirth. In fact it is good to remember once again that your labor and delivery will involve teamwork between you and your husband and between you and your physician. The performance or nonperformance of an episiotomy will be entirely your doctor's responsibility, though you should discuss your ideas and feelings about this process with your doctor, and you should know what you can do to acquire good control of your pelvic floor muscles to help yourself and the doctor. Practice of the Kegel exercises at least 20–30 times a day will make your pelvic floor muscles more flexible. I would also suggest a daily massage of the pelvic floor using any soft ointment.

THE THIRD STAGE OF LABOR

The third stage of labor is the expulsion of the afterbirth or "placenta." Once the baby has been born, the doctor will clamp and cut the umbilical cord. This procedure does not hurt either you or your baby. A few minutes after the birth of your child your uterus will contract again and your doctor will ask you to push once more to expel the placenta. He/she will generally help you by exerting pressure on your abdomen. The expulsion of the placenta is generally very fast, taking only a few minutes.

This has been our first class. For the next session I would like you to wear shorts, tights, slacks or any comfortable garment that will allow you to perform our exercises easily. We will continue to look at these pictures and discuss the process of labor in more detail. I will never teach an exercise by itself, but will always explain—with the help of these pictures—why we perform certain exercises during each phase of labor.

LESSON 2

Learning to relax and conserve your energy through neuromuscular control exercises; simple but basic exercises to prepare your body for childbirth.

This lesson will be a more active one for you and your husband. We are going to do exercises today, which I divide into two groups:

1. Neuromuscular control exercises, which I also call Concentration-Relaxation exercises.

2. Stretch or limbering exercises.

One of the primary aims during labor must be the conservation of energy. You should never exert more energy than is actually needed for efficient performance during this period. By conserving energy you will avoid unnecessary fatigue. If you are tense, if you thrash around or dig your fingernails into the mattress (or your partner's arm), you are wasting energy.

NEUROMUSCULAR CONTROL EXERCISES

Neuromuscular control exercises are extremely important. You must remember that the uterus will be working hard during labor. That part of your body will be extremely active. Your task will be to allow it to work freely while you keep the rest of your body deliberately relaxed. These exercises will help you to develop muscle control, to isolate muscle groups, and at the same time make you aware of which muscle groups are in use and which are at rest.

These exercises will have to be practiced with your partner. Not only is it impossible for you to check on your own relaxation, but I want your partner to give the commands, which I will demonstrate. I also want him to check on your tension and relaxation. In this way you will learn to react to your partner's signals instantly, and he will learn to recognize any tensions in your body. You will be involved in labor and may not notice that while trying to control the uterine contractions, you have tensed your legs or arms or face. Your partner, however, will see these tensions immediately, and you will be able to cooperate and relax whenever he gives the signal. I think the great advantage of your working together is that since you have shared your lives for some time, you know each other very well, and are therefore much more aware of each other's tensions and difficulties than a strange nurse or doctor could ever be. And this intimate knowledge can be used in working together in labor and correcting tensions. I am often sure that I can tell what kind of day my husband has had when he comes home, even before he has said a word. It's his facial expression, perhaps, or the way he holds his shoulders. I'm not even sure what it is. Try it sometime with your partner. Watch him or her, and soon you'll be able to spot tensions and weak points. This will make it easier to react to each other's signals.

This exercise will require considerable discipline from both of you. Your partner's commands have to be as disciplined as your reaction. By developing this kind of teamwork, it will be easy for you to react to his signals, even under stress.

Sit comfortably on a chair; your shoulders, arms and feet well supported. A pillow under your knees will help relax your legs. Also be sure to separate your legs so that they gently rotate out when you relax them. I prefer you to practice relaxation in the sitting position, as lying on your back may be very uncomfortable, given the baby's weight. Sitting or lying on your side may be more comfortable. Some women even find it impossible to

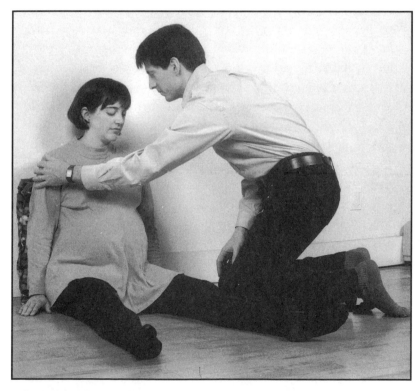

Phil is helping Sue to relax.

lie on their back, as the baby is pressing on their main vein and artery and this may make them feel faint.

Begin by taking a very deep and relaxing inhalation-exhalation. I call such a deep relaxing breath "a cleansing breath." From now on, when I speak of a "cleansing breath," you will know that I want you to take a deep breath, then exhale and relax your whole body. Your partner should now check your relaxation. Let him gently lift your arm by holding your wrist in his hand and feeling the whole weight of your arm and shoulder. Let your arm bend at the elbow so that every joint is relaxed. Once your partner feels the weight of your arm, he can then try to move your arm freely from side to side to check on your absolute relaxation. When he lets go of your arm, it should drop heavily down. Let him try your other arm. To check the relaxation of your legs, your partner must place his hands under your knees and gently bend them a little. If your leg is tense, he will not be able to bend your knee easily and he should therefore remind you to relax.

Once your partner is satisfied that you are relaxed, he should give the following command: "Contract your right arm." You will then tense your arm, shoulder, elbow, fist, and raise your arm, holding it straight before you, at shoulder level. Your partner should check on the tension in your right arm, then check on the complete relaxation of your left arm and both legs—while you are still holding up your right arm. The command is: "Release your arm," and your arm should fall down absolutely relaxed.

Command: "Contract your left arm." Tense the arm, shoulder, elbow, fist, and raise your left arm, holding it straight before you, at shoulder level. Again your partner should check first on the tension in your left arm and then, while the left arm is

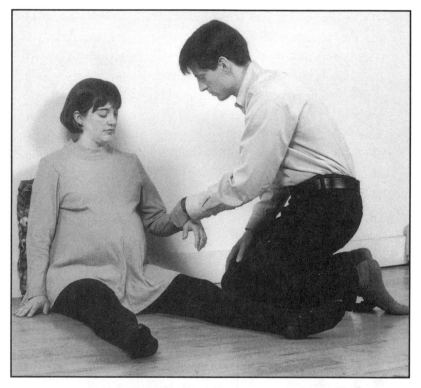

Phil and Sue begin the neuromuscular control exercises. Note complete relaxation of her neck, face, arms and legs.

tense, he must check on the relaxation of your right arm and both your legs. Next command: "Release your left arm."

Command: "Contract your right leg." Stiffen your thigh, hold the leg straight and flex your foot. You don't have to raise your leg. While you are holding your leg stiff, your partner should check first on the tension of the right leg, then on the relaxation of your left leg and both arms, checking your shoulders and face at the same time. Command: "Release your leg."

Command: "Contract right arm, right leg." Again your part-

ner will check on your tension on the right side and your
release of muscles on your left. "Release."

Command: "Contract left arm, left leg." Be sure to stiffen
your leg well and to flex your foot in order to tense the calf
muscles. Your partner will check your tension and relaxation.
"Release."

Command: "Contract your right arm, left leg." Your partner
will check and give the command: "Release."

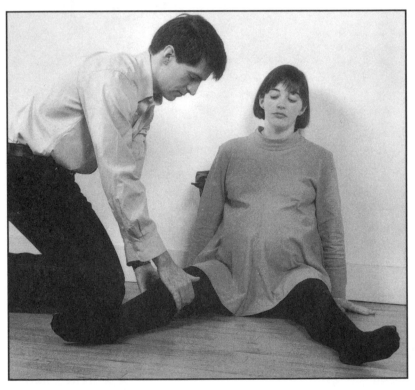

Phil checks relaxation on Sue's right leg.

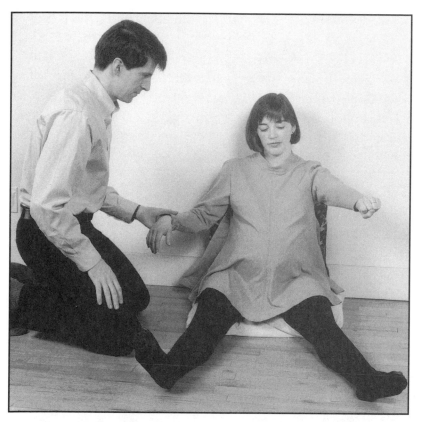

Sue is contracting her left arm and right leg, while Phil is checking relaxation in her right arm and left leg.

Command: "Contract your left arm, right leg." Your partner will check and release.

You will soon realize how very difficult it is to work with one part of your body while keeping the rest of your body relaxed. It will demand your absolute concentration and special attention. You will discover that only with continued and repeated practice will you be able to isolate muscle groups and automatically follow your partner's signals. You should practice these exercises at least once a day. You will soon find that the two of you will develop your own way of working together: Gentle touch, a stroking of a tense part, verbal, or often non-verbal communication between you.

Let me point out once again that the purpose of these exercises is to make you aware of your body, to establish a

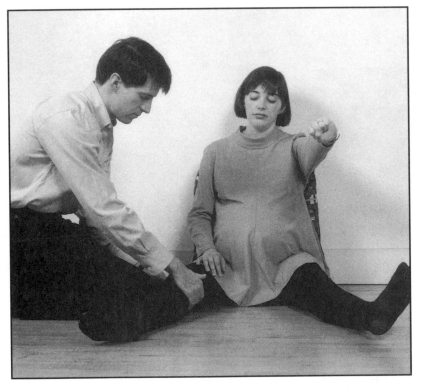

Now Sue is contracting her left arm and left leg, and Phil is checking relaxation in her right leg.

source of teamwork between you and your partner and to enable you to be economical with all energy expended during labor. You realize, of course, that you won't tense and lift an arm in labor, or tense a leg. This exercise is a training for labor, to make you become aware of your body and thus able to separate muscle groups, relaxing part of your body as other parts are working. At the same time, it will allow your partner to become aware and recognize your tensions and allow him to find ways and means to help and correct.

Relaxation, combined with the breathing, is the most important aspect of your whole training for childbirth. None of the breathing techniques will really help you, unless you are able to let your body relax and thus help the uterus to do its work to open the passage for your baby.

STRETCH AND LIMBERING EXERCISES

I think we all tend to slow down considerably during pregnancy, partly because of the added weight we have to carry, partly because of our own anxiety that we might somehow injure the baby when we stretch, bend or simply move around. So many people shower us with well-meant advice not to do this, that or the other. I am sure you have been told by someone not to reach or raise your arms above your head, not to cross your legs, etc. If we really followed all this well-intended counsel, we could hardly move at all.

It is perfectly safe to lead a normal life and to move about as much as you have always done, as long as it does not hurt and you don't get too tired. I always like to quote Dr. Alan Guttmacher here. He told us once that as a young obstetrician he used to forbid his patients to play tennis, though he allowed every other sport. In discussing this with a colleague, the colleague said, "Strange, I forbid my patients to go swimming and allow them to do anything else!" They realized that they were both discouraging the particular sport they themselves didn't like or were poor at.

The stretch and limbering exercises I will show you are meant to make you feel better now. They will strengthen your back and abdominal muscles so you can carry the additional weight of the baby with comparative ease. They will help you to spread your legs far apart, which will be most useful for you when you have to push out your baby. Some of the exercises will improve the tone of your pelvic-floor muscles.

For the following exercises you do not need a pillow under your head or knees. And don't practice any of these exercises on your bed, even if you think your mattress is very hard. The hardest mattress is still too soft. You need firm support. Use the floor, covered by a rug or blanket.

Exercise 1: Sit cross-legged (tailor fashion) on the floor, back relaxed and slightly rounded. Use this sitting position as much as possible from now on. It will help to strengthen your pelvic-floor muscles and stretch your thigh muscles. We rarely sit in this position any more, with all our comfortable upholstered chairs and couches. I suggest you do this in the evenings while you read, sew, watch television or play chess with your husband. When you get tired of sitting like this, stretch your legs for a while, shake them out, then resume the position.

Exercise 2: Sit on the floor and put the soles of your feet together, then pull your feet as close to your body as possible. Put your hands on your thighs and press them gently down. You

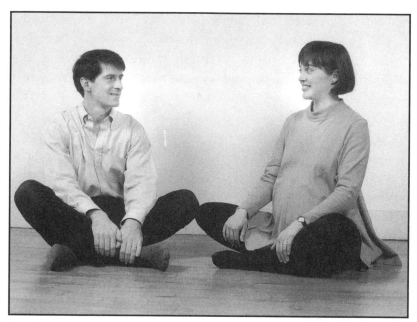

Exercise 1

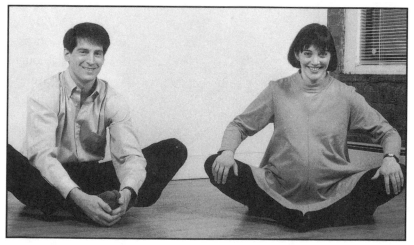

Exercise 2

will feel the muscles pull on the inside of your thighs. For those of you who have very long ligaments, this exercise may be very easy. Your thighs will practically touch the floor with little effort. If so, try the following exercise: Sit on the floor, stretch your legs well apart and turn your knees out. Then lean your body forward, and you will feel a good pull in your thighs.

Exercise 3: Extend your legs to stretch your pelvis and your thighs.

Exercise 4: The spinal stretch. Sit cross-legged or with the soles of your feet together. Inhale—then exhale and raise your arms above your head, looking at your fingertips—reaching with each arm and breathing in and out. Repeat 3 to 5 times with each arm.

Exercise 5: Sit straight. Raise your arms to shoulder level as you inhale. Take your left arm to the left and look over your left shoulder as you exhale. Inhale and bring left arm to center.

Exercise 3

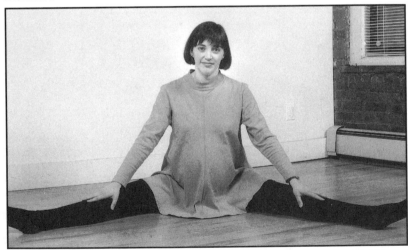

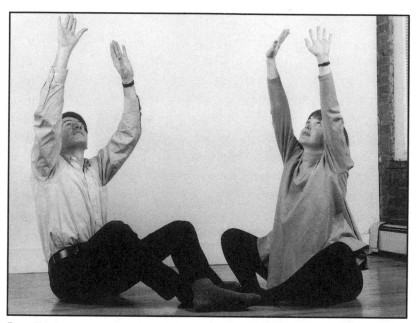

Exercise 4

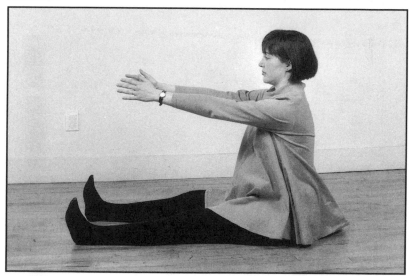

Exercise 5

Exhale and stretch right arm back, looking over your right shoulder. Inhale and bring the arm back to center. Repeat 3 times with each arm. Do not forget to breathe.

Exercise 6: Exhale. Round your back, lower your head and tighten your buttocks. This exercise strengthens your lower back and increases mobility in your spine. Repeat 4 times.

Exercise 7: Lie on your back, knees bent, knees and feet hip-width apart. Inhale. Slowly raise your back and buttocks off the floor. Exhale. Lower your back slowly to the floor vertebra by vertebra. Repeat from the straight position. Inhale and raise your buttocks and back. Exhale and slowly lower your back to the floor. Repeat 3 times.

Exercise 5

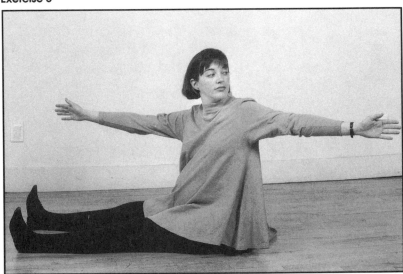

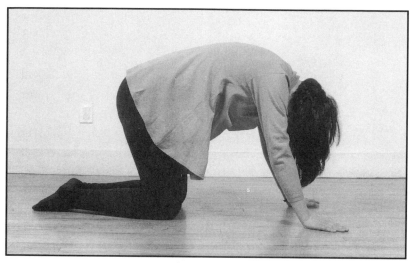

Exercise 6

Exerciso 7

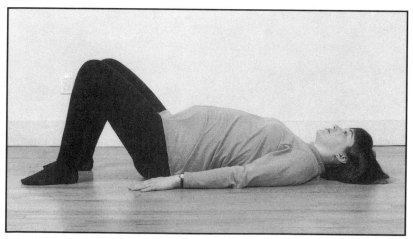

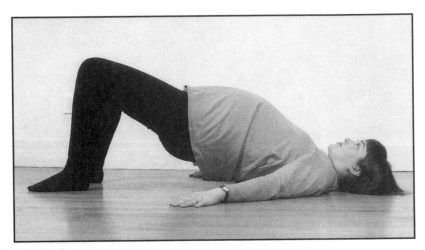

Exercise 7

Exercise 7

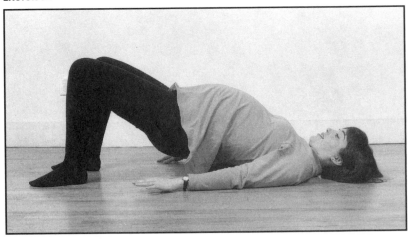

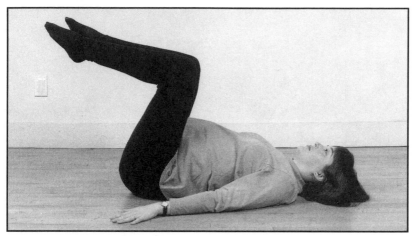

Exercise 8

Exercise 8: To rise from the floor: Bend both legs off the floor. Slowly drop both legs to one side. Support your body with arm and knee. Come back to the sitting position. Getting up in this way will avoid strain on your abdominal muscles and your back.

Exercise 8

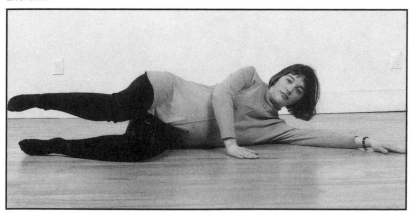

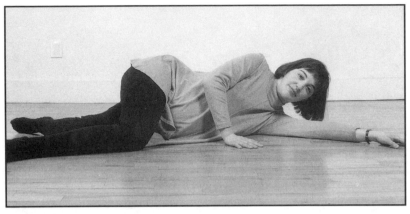

Exercise 8

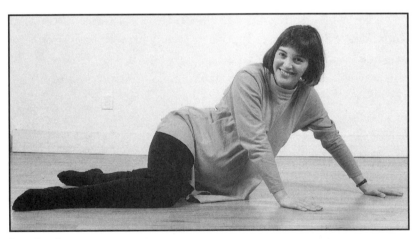

Exercise 8

Be sure to practice these exercises daily with your partner, so that he can supervise and correct you, and so that both of you can understand the purpose of our first two groups of exercises.

We will start with our third group of exercises, respiration exercises, in the next lesson.

LESSON 3

*Three phases of uterine contractions:
latent, accelerated, transitional;
our first breathing technique; partner's
role during practice at home.*

It is always important to review the material covered in our previous lesson. These reviews are an essential aspect of your training. Not that I don't trust you to practice diligently, but it is imperative to see how proficient you have become, and to correct a few things that you may have misunderstood. Therefore bear with me when I encourage you to repeat and repeat the exercises. This is the discipline of the Lamaze technique. You will have to learn to channel your energy correctly for your labor, and I will help you do so.

Let us review the neuromuscular control exercises. Do you remember what these are for? Do we actually tense one arm or leg in labor? Certainly not. These exercises will teach you to relax part of your body while the rest is working, and they will also help to establish teamwork between you and your partner. Sit comfortably, take a deep "cleansing breath" and relax. Let your partner check your relaxation before he gives the commands.

Then: Contract right arm. Release. Contract left arm (partner should check thoroughly). Release. Contract right arm and right leg (partner checks). Release. Contract left arm and left leg (partner checks). Release. Contract right arm and left leg (partner checks). Release. Contract left arm and right leg (partner checks). Release. Review the exercise once more in the sitting position.

I hope you will notice how much you have improved in one week. It should be much easier for you to isolate muscle groups and to follow your partner's commands. Some of you will learn faster than others, but in a relatively short time you will have learned this difficult body control. Remember also that it is really a good idea to have this control whether you are pregnant or not. I use the relaxation in long plane rides, by discovering tensions in my body and deliberately releasing those parts—thus avoiding a great deal of fatigue.

Now let us review the stretch and limbering exercises. These can be done without your partner's help, though he may enjoy doing them with you. It is often more fun to exercise in company. Sit on the floor cross-legged. Then put the soles of your feet together, your hands on your thighs, and press your thighs gently down.

Extend your legs to stretch your pelvis and thighs.

Sit straight. Raise your arms to shoulder level as you inhale. Take your left arm to the left and look over your left shoulder as you exhale. Inhale and bring left arm to center. Exhale and stretch right arm back looking over your right shoulder. Inhale and bring the arm back to center. Repeat 3 times with each arm. Do not forget to breathe.

Exhale. Round your back, lower your head and tighten your

buttocks. This exercise strengthens your lower back and increases mobility in your spine. Repeat 4 times.

Lie on your back, bend your knees, feet firmly on the floor, heels close to your buttocks. Inhale and slowly raise your back off the floor, hips toward the ceiling, then exhale slowly as you lower your back vertebra by vertebra and rest your back.

Here is the last exercise: the spinal stretch. Sit cross-legged, bend your arms to your shoulders, then stretch them well into the air. Look at your fingertips, stretch a little more, and a little more, and a little more. Then relax and breathe deeply. You will find it feels wonderful to be able to stretch, and you can rest assured that it will not do you or the baby any harm whatsoever.

If any of you have been to physical fitness or dance classes, you will probably be able to think of other suitable exercises. Be sure, however, never to raise or lower both legs at the same time when you are lying flat on your back.

THE THREE PHASES OF THE FIRST STAGE OF LABOR

I want you to look once again at the pictures and drawings showing the first stage of labor. You will remember that the first stage of labor consists of the effacement—or thinning out and flattening—of the cervix, and its dilation to 5 fingers or 10 centimeters.

We divide the first stage of labor into three parts or phases.

Part One is the *latent* or *preliminary* phase of labor, during which the cervix effaces fully and dilates to about 1^{1}/2 fingers or 3 centimeters.

Part Two is the dilation of the cervix from about 1½ fingers or 3 centimeters to approximately 4 fingers or 8 centimeters. This phase is called the *accelerated,* or *active* phase of labor.

Part Three is the dilation of the cervix from 4 fingers to full dilation or 5 fingers or, in centimeters, from 8 to 10. This phase is called the *transition* phase.

The uterine contractions change their character in the three phases of the first stage of labor. The uterus, like any other muscle in our body, contracts and relaxes. This is the nature of muscle. Stretch your arm out, then bend it slowly. In doing this, you have used a muscle—that is, you have contracted the biceps. When you straighten your arm again you release the tension in the biceps. Suppose you were to draw a diagram of a muscular contraction; it would look like a curve, or a wave pattern.

Look at the diagrams on page 62, which will show you the changes in the waves that occur during the three phases of the first stage of labor. I like to compare these waves to those at the oceanside. There are many people, and you may be among them, who can surf very well, meeting each wave with confidence and riding with it and through it. And then there are people like myself: I don't know how to cope with these waves. Should I face them? Should my back be turned toward them? And before I have managed to make up my mind, the wave has hit me, thrown me over. I scrape my knees, get water in my mouth and nose and scramble out exhausted, telling myself not to try again until the next summer.

I think one can compare the trained or untrained woman in labor to the person who has learned or who has not learned to ride the waves at the beach.

A few years ago, though, a friend showed me how to manage the waves when we were swimming together, and though I never became an expert at it, I could manage to ride, if not most, at least many of the waves—and I felt very good about it. Even if I missed one, I was confident that I could cope with the next one. And so it is in labor: you probably won't catch every wave; you'll goof occasionally, but you will stay on top of most of them, and you will say as one of my students said, "It actually got easier and easier the more labor progressed, because I got better and better." Another of my students told me, "The fact that I could participate in the birth of my child and knew what to do and actively give birth was the greatest ego trip I've ever had in my life!"

In the *preliminary* or *latent phase* of labor (1) the waves are gentle and shallow. One wave may last from 30 to 45 seconds, and the intervals of rest may vary from 5 to 20 minutes. This first phase of labor, where the contractions are mild, lasts quite a long time. A study of the labor of many women has shown that the average time may be about 8 to 9 hours. For most of this period you will probably be at home, and you won't even need any breathing control for a great part of this phase.

If you are one of those very rare women who do have extremely easy and fast labors, you may not need every step of our training. But I would much rather have you prepare yourself for the average: a normal, lengthy labor. Should labor be faster than you anticipated, you will find that you are prepared to cope. For second or third babies, the average time limits for the three phases of the first stage of labor will be about half those of the first. Your actual contractions will feel the same, but the whole labor will be telescoped.

3 PHASES OF FIRST STAGE OF LABOR

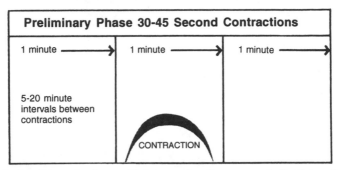

Preliminary Phase 30-45 Second Contractions

1 minute ⟶   1 minute ⟶   1 minute ⟶

5-20 minute
intervals between
contractions

CONTRACTION

1. During this early phase of labor, contractions occur in the form of mild waves that come at irregular intervals.

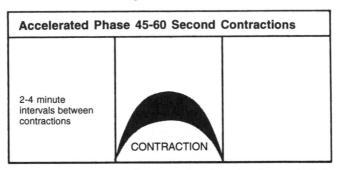

Accelerated Phase 45-60 Second Contractions

2-4 minute
intervals between
contractions

CONTRACTION

2. The accelerated phase is the longest and most active period of labor. Waves become higher and last longer.

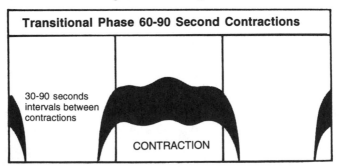

Transitional Phase 60-90 Second Contractions

30-90 seconds
intervals between
contractions

CONTRACTION

3. This phase is the most intense and the shortest phase of the first stage of labor. Waves are erratic and sharp.

During the second, or *accelerated phase*, the waves of uterine contractions are higher, as you can see from the diagram, and the intervals between the contractions have shortened considerably. The length of one wave may be from 45 to 60 seconds by now, and the periods of rest are shorter, usually from 2 to 4 minutes.

The same study of the labor of many women has shown that the average length of time for the accelerated phase—the dilation of the cervix from about 3 to 8 centimeters or $1^1/_2$ to 4 fingers—is about 3 to 4 hours.

The *transition* is the third phase of the first stage of labor. The contractions, represented as waves in our diagram, have become long, strong and erratic. They may have several peaks. They build up to maximum strength very quickly. They may last up to $1^1/_2$ minutes, and the intervals between contractions are now shorter than the contractions themselves. The interval of rest may only be from 30 seconds to about 90 seconds. In fact, you may have just congratulated yourself that you managed to get through one of these contractions when you feel the next one already beginning. This, as you can imagine, is the hardest part of your labor. The only saving grace is that this phase is the shortest of the three subdivisions of the first stage of labor, and will usually last only from half an hour to an hour. I don't want to minimize the severity of the transitional contractions. You should be prepared for them and you should realize that this is like the final sprint of the uterine muscles. This period will demand more concentrated effort than any part previously experienced. But I will give you tools to work with and teach you how best to cope with this difficult part of your labor. One of my students reported to me one day on her labor.

She said, "You talked of waves in labor, but it was a hurricane that hit me in transition."

The reason that I have given you approximate time limits for these phases of labor is to let you have some idea of what to expect. I cannot emphasize enough, however, that these are averages. There are many variations, all within the norm, and I want you to realize that it is very unlikely that your labor will be like any textbook description. Do not let this disturb you. In fact, it is one of the great advantages of the Lamaze technique that it provides the techniques to use as your individual labor demands. No two labors are the same. Even your own subsequent labors will differ and change in character from delivery to delivery.

THE FIRST TECHNIQUE OF BREATHING FOR THE FIRST STAGE OF LABOR

I will now give you three different breathing techniques to use during your first stage of labor. As you pass from preliminary labor, through accelerated labor, to the transition, you will adjust your breathing to the changes of the uterine contractions. I always think of this as if I were driving a car, shifting from first to second to third gear. It would never occur to you to stay in first gear when you want to go faster. In the same way, you will have to "shift gears" as your labor progresses, in order to stay in control of your uterine contractions.

And now to the first breathing technique you will use in early labor. Be sure not to use this technique as long as you can walk, talk or laugh through a contraction. You may get so

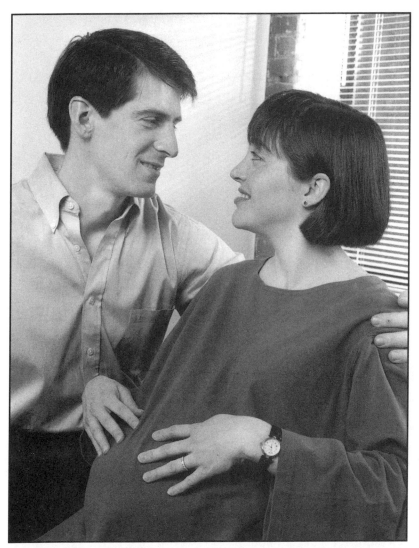

To begin breathing practice, focus on fixed object, breathe in through nose, out through mouth, massage abdomen.

excited at the onset of your labor that you will want to breathe with it even if there is no actual need. Please don't, because you will soon become very bored by the whole process. Remember that the first phase can take hours and hours. You'd be better off going for a walk with your husband, seeing a movie or tending to your usual house activities. We often get so excited at the onset of labor that we want to rush off to the hospital, hoping the baby will come quicker once we are there. Time, on the contrary, will seem endless if you arrive at the hospital too early. There is little in the labor or birthing room to divert your attention, and you may find this very demoralizing. At home, you will be more relaxed and fortified with the confidence your training has given you to handle the long latent part of labor. Of course, your own physician will give you exact instructions as to when he wants to be called. But my general advice is, don't rush.

Our aim during labor is to create a strong center of concentration through disciplined activity. The breathing technique we use has to be deliberate and different from our normal automatic breathing. I want you to breathe with your chest. Try it first by placing your hands flat under your breasts and letting your middle fingers meet. When you breathe with your chest, you will notice that your middle fingers will part slightly when you inhale and come together again when you exhale. Keep your abdomen relaxed while you breathe in this fashion. To make this chest breathing even more deliberate, I want you to inhale through your nose and exhale through your mouth. It's almost like whistling the air out. Take from 6 to 9 breaths in a minute, and count your breaths as you practice.

Begin every contraction by taking a deep cleansing breath. This will give you a good exchange of oxygen and carbon dioxide at the onset of a contraction, and at the same time

BREATHING EXERCISES FOR FIRST STAGE OF LABOR

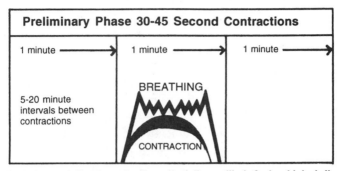

Preliminary Phase 30-45 Second Contractions

1 minute ⟶ 1 minute ⟶ 1 minute ⟶

5-20 minute intervals between contractions

BREATHING

CONTRACTION

1. **Begin wave with cleansing breath, follow with 6-9 chest inhalation-exhalations, conclude with cleansing breath.**

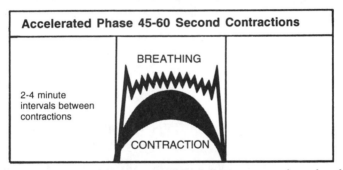

Accelerated Phase 45-60 Second Contractions

2-4 minute intervals between contractions

BREATHING

CONTRACTION

2. **Take cleansing breath; accelerate breathing as wave rises, decelerate as it subsides; finish with a cleansing breath.**

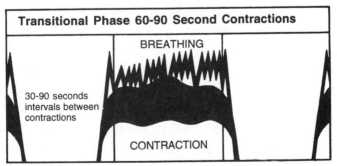

Transitional Phase 60-90 Second Contractions

30-90 seconds intervals between contractions

BREATHING

CONTRACTION

3. **Take cleansing breath; continue pattern of 4-6 breaths, then a short blowing out; take a final cleansing breath.**

relax you. Relaxation is a most important factor, as our usual reaction to a uterine contraction is what is called a "flight reaction." We tense our whole body. By taking a cleansing breath at the beginning of each contraction, you begin the contraction in a relaxed condition.

Now inhale through your nose, exhale through your lips, making a little noise with your breathing in order to keep a good rhythm. Count your breaths, and end each contraction with another cleansing breath and smile. The relaxing breath and smile at the end of each contraction is also of great importance. It means that you really come to a full stop, at the end of each contraction, emotionally and physically. The smile is intended to help you relax. As you know, a tense person rarely smiles. Once the muscles of your face are relaxed, it is more likely that the rest of your body will relax, as well.

WHAT TO DO WITH YOUR HANDS

It's very difficult to know what to do with one's hands in labor. You certainly should not grip the sides of your bed or dig your fingernails into your husband's arm. In order to avoid such tension, do what comes naturally and soothe the pain by massaging your abdomen gently in time to your breathing. This is the best way to do it: Cupping your hands lightly, place them under your abdomen. Then massage gently with your fingertips, leading your arms out and up while you inhale, completing the circle down again as you exhale. This massage, or "effleurage" as it is called professionally, not only provides another point of concentration, but also feels good. A light massage will help to relieve the tension in your abdomen during a contraction. It actually has the same effect as rubbing a place on your body that hurts. You can also try to massage your abdomen with one hand, using your whole hand gently. Or you may like to let your partner gently massage your belly. He can sit at your side and, using the palm of his hand, massage your abdomen slowly.

If you have to use a fetal monitor, which requires two belts around your belly, one for monitoring the fetal heart, the other for monitoring the uterine contraction, it will be difficult to use your hands in a circular movement over your abdomen. However, you will find that a gentle massage just over the lowest part of your abdomen will feel very soothing. It may happen that your abdomen becomes so sensitive in labor, that you cannot stand either your own hand or your partner's. In that case ask him or her to massage your back gently in a circular motion. The coach should keep his/her fingers together, cup the hand slightly and massage the back soothingly.

HYPERVENTILATION

Occasionally you may feel a little dizzy when you practice this deliberate breathing technique. We call this hyperventilation, or what happens when the balance between the oxygen intake and the carbon dioxide output is disturbed. During a prolonged practice session you may even feel a tingling or stiffening in your hands and feet or around your lips. It is unlikely, however, that this will happen in labor, as your uterus will need a great deal of oxygen while it is contracting. But just in case, here are two easy ways to overcome this: Cup your hands, hold them over your nose and mouth and breathe in your own carbon dioxide; or hold your breath for a few seconds when the contraction is over. This will soon accumulate enough carbon dioxide, and your dizziness will quickly disappear. Hyperventilation is most likely to occur in labor during the *accelerated* and *transition* stages. I suggest that if you become hyperventilated at the hospital and do not want to hold your breath, use a little paper sandwich bag to breathe into. This will be more effective than using your hands. And since you are going to bring this little paper bag along, there are a few things you can add to it which may be useful during labor. One of these is a small can of talcum powder. In actual labor you will be massaging your skin during each contraction. Your fingers may get hot and sticky. You may irritate your abdomen after a long period of massaging. Use the talcum powder on your abdomen or your hands to avoid such excessive friction. Let your partner sprinkle it on whenever you need it. You could also use a soft lotion to massage your abdomen. (Later we'll discover many other things to carry along in our Lamaze bag.)

Keep your eyes open during a contraction and while practicing the breathing technique. Be sure, however, to focus on one point in the room. This will help you to concentrate. You will find that nothing happening outside your line of vision will concern you. It is vitally important to maintain this discipline in your practice session since during real labor you will need every ounce of concentration. An even better way would be to have eye contact with your partner. He could then work easily with you and correct your breathing when necessary. You may find that in practicing the eye contact with him, you'll probably break up laughing. But to tell the truth, I've never seen anybody laugh or giggle through labor, though I must admit that would be a great way to have a baby!

POSITION OF BODY DURING
EARLY LABOR

You do not have to lie down when you are in labor. We always assume that the moment we go into the hospital we have to lie down in a bed and behave like a sick person. I want you to remember that having a baby is a healthy event, and that the only reason we go to a hospital is because it is safer, not because we are suffering from a disease. I realize it isn't easy to overcome the notion that hospitals are places where one must suffer.

It is interesting to remember that over fifty years ago, when most women delivered their babies at home, nobody would have thought to call a laboring woman "a patient." She was just "a woman in labor" or "a woman giving birth to her child." It was only when women were encouraged to have their babies in hospitals that the laboring woman was called a "patient," a term that obviously makes us think of illness and suffering.

In fact, with the introduction of the episiotomy (a small surgical incision in the area between vagina and anus to allow the baby to emerge more easily and without tearing), having a baby actually became a surgical procedure.

In the labor room you will be asked to undress and put on a hospital gown, which is usually not attractive at all. I know you would much rather wear your own pretty gown. But remember that this hospital gown is functional, serves a good purpose and is far more practical to wear during labor than your own. On the other hand, if you would feel better in your own gown, don't hesitate to tell your doctor or midwife.

When the attending nurse asks you to get into bed, you will

see a bed (with usually just one pillow) higher than your own for the convenience of doctors and nurses. It is narrow with bars on both sides, which you can use to support yourself. Don't forget that all hospital beds can be rolled up. Ask your nurse to roll it to any angle that is comfortable. Most of us can breathe better with our backs and heads raised, or even sitting up, and there is no reason you should not experiment in order to find your own comfortable position. You may want to lie on your side. The left side is recommended, because your main artery and vein are located a little to the right, and by lying on your left side you do not compress your aorta or vena cava and deprive your baby of oxygen. Sit up tailor fashion, legs crossed, or recline at any angle that suits you. You will only have to lie flat when you are being examined or when your physician suggests a certain position that he prefers you to be in. It may be a good idea to bring a couple of pillows to the hospital in order to be comfortable. I would suggest, however, that you put some colored pillowcases on them so that they won't be pushed into the laundry bag with all the hospital linen.

Most hospitals are now offering "birthing rooms" or "single room maternity care." Birthing rooms vary from labor rooms by frequently being cheerfully furnished, but mainly by offering a "birthing bed," which can be easily taken apart when you enter your pushing stage, so that your legs are lower than your buttocks. Well supported, you can sit upright, and you can push your baby out in a more "physiological" position, i.e., from above down, instead of lying prone with your legs raised in stirrups.

The single room maternity care allows a woman not only to labor and deliver in one room and bed, but also spend her postpartum period there, without having to be moved to a different room for the length of her stay in the hospital.

PARTNER'S ROLE DURING PRACTICE

When you practice the first breathing technique at home, let your partner give you precise commands. He should have a stop watch with a sweep second hand to time you. Practice the breathing for approximately one minute—occasionally varying the time from 40 to 60 seconds to imitate the length of a real contraction. It is extremely important that your partner be as precise in his commands as you will have to be in your performance. Therefore he has to give the command: *contraction begins* and then *contraction ends*, and not just say "start" and "stop." This is important because you are training yourself to react to a uterine contraction with a respiratory response instead of a flight response. We are using therefore what is called "secondary conditioning," which means the correct command has to trigger your reaction.

It will also be helpful if your partner calls off the seconds while you practice your breathing. He should say: "Contraction begins," and then call out, "15 seconds . . . 30 seconds . . . 45 seconds . . . contraction ends." You will find this a very helpful device. It will make the contraction seem shorter. When your partner calls out 30 seconds, you will know that you are at the halfway point and when he says 45 seconds, it will mean "going, going, going, gone." Many couples find this not only useful during practice sessions, but also in actual labor. Your partner's signal at that time will be your cleansing breath. From

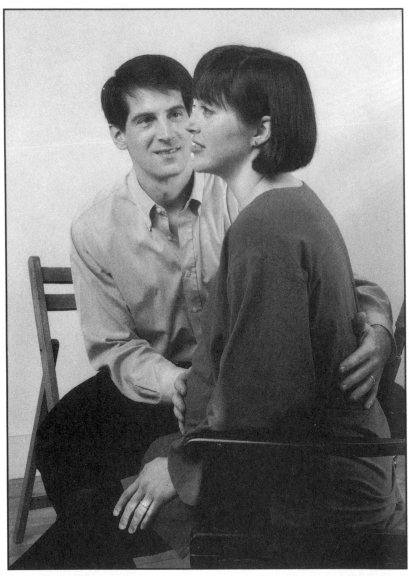

It is both important and helpful for the partner to supervise his partner while she practices her breathing.

this he will know that you have started another contraction. He will then look at his watch and call out the seconds for you. Try it and see how you like it.

Now let's practice the first breathing technique. Take up any position that is comfortable for you. Contraction begins. Take a deep, relaxing, cleansing breath. Breathe in through your nose, and slowly exhale through your lips. Count your breaths, focus your eyes on a point in the room, or even better have eye contact with your partner, and massage your abdomen lightly with your fingertips, out and up as you inhale, down as you exhale. Or let your partner gently massage your abdomen or your back. Finish with a deep cleansing breath and a smile. Be sure to keep the rest of your body as relaxed as possible while practicing.

When you practice by yourself, give yourself commands—contraction begins, contraction ends—and follow the time on a clock with a second hand. Also visualize the pictures and diagrams that show contractions, so that it will be clear in your mind how your body is working at the time. It always helps to imagine the wave of a contraction and how you will ride the wave with your breathing technique. And be sure to practice your breathing with any Braxton-Hicks contraction* that you may feel.

---

* Braxton-Hicks contractions are actual uterine contractions, which become noticeable the closer you come to the end of your pregnancy. They are generally not painful, though you will feel a distinct tightening of your abdomen. Toward the end of your pregnancy they may, hopefully, have started effacing the cervix and perhaps even dilating it a little.

LESSON 4

What to do for back labor; breathing techniques two and three, for the accelerated and transitional phases; how the partner can simulate a contraction.

We will begin by reviewing what you have learned in the previous lessons. I expect you to carry on with the neuromuscular control exercises, so you can improve your body control and you and your partner can develop good teamwork. I am sure you will have noticed by now that the body building and stretch exercises are no longer so tiring. In fact, you probably feel better for performing them and strengthening these muscles that have to carry most of the strain during pregnancy.

And now again to our first breathing technique. Do you think that by now you can describe our first technique to a friend who has never heard of it? You would have to begin by telling her that we divide the first stage of labor into three parts. They are: 1) The preliminary or latent part of labor, in which the cervix effaces and starts to dilate. 2) The accelerated part of labor, in which the cervix dilates approximately from 3 to 8 centimeters, or $1\frac{1}{2}$ to 4 fingers. And, finally 3) The transition, in which the cervix dilates from approximately 8 to 10 centimeters, or 4 to 5 fingers. The waves of uterine contractions change in character as labor progresses, and you will remember that you must synchronize your breathing techniques with the intensity of the sensations that you will feel.

Then you must tell your friend what the actual breathing technique is like. We begin the contraction by taking a deep, relaxing, cleansing breath. This is followed by deliberate chest breathing, inhaling through the nose, exhaling through the mouth. We finish, when the contraction subsides, with another deep, relaxing, cleansing breath and a smile. We take any position that is comfortable, concentrating on one point in the room or having eye contact. At the same time we effleurage, or massage, our abdomen, moving our fingertips lightly in a circular motion to the rhythm of our breathing, or we encourage our partner to massage our abdomen gently.

Now try the breathing once again while I give the commands: Contraction begins. Take a deep, cleansing breath. Now breathe comfortably and deliberately with your chest, inhale through your nose, exhale through your mouth, 15 seconds, 30 seconds, 45 seconds . . . the contraction is over. End with a deep cleansing breath and a smile. Did you have between 6 and 9 breaths during this simulated contraction?

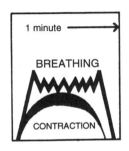

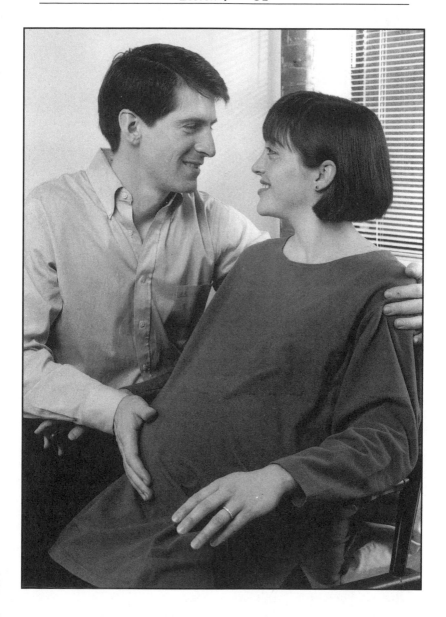

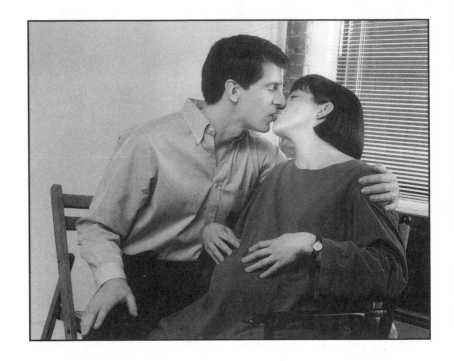

WHERE DO YOU FEEL A CONTRACTION?

I wonder if you have ever thought about where in your abdomen you will actually feel a contraction? Will you feel it all over, just low down, or perhaps in the back? Actually, the majority of women feel their labor low down, just above the pubic bone, but deep inside and spreading toward the groin. Some may feel a contraction beginning in the lower back and radiating to the lower abdomen, even drawing into the thighs. If you feel your labor in your legs, massage your legs! Don't get stuck rubbing your belly when most of the pain is in your thighs. Remember, I give you the tools to work with, but it will be up to you, according to your labor, to decide how and when you use the tools. All this demands a great flexibility on your part, but it also makes sense that you react to your body and its own rhythm instead of to what I have said or what you may have read in a textbook.

I remember being woken one morning by a telephone call. An excited voice was saying, "Mrs. Bing, Mrs. Bing, we are in the hospital and it's all in Charlotte's legs! What can we do?" I managed to open my eyes and say sleepily, "Massage her thighs." "Oh," said the voice on the other end of the line. Then I heard a click and I could see in my mind how he was racing upstairs to massage Charlotte's thighs. About twenty-five percent of woman experience what is called "back labor." I want you all to be aware of the fact that back labor exists. I am sure this may come as a surprise for many of you. After all, why should one feel anything in the back, when one imagines that the uterus is right there in front in the abdomen? Obviously the baby is there in front too, and the most natural thing would be to expect labor where one imagines the baby and uterus to be.

There is no one cause for back labor. However, it most often occurs when the baby lies in a posterior position: the baby is facing the mother's abdomen with the back of his head pressed against her spine. It is important, therefore, for you to be prepared for a possible experience of back labor.

WAYS TO ALLEVIATE BACK LABOR

Now what can we do about back labor? Your breathing technique should remain the same, whether you feel contractions in your abdomen or in your back. However, it is

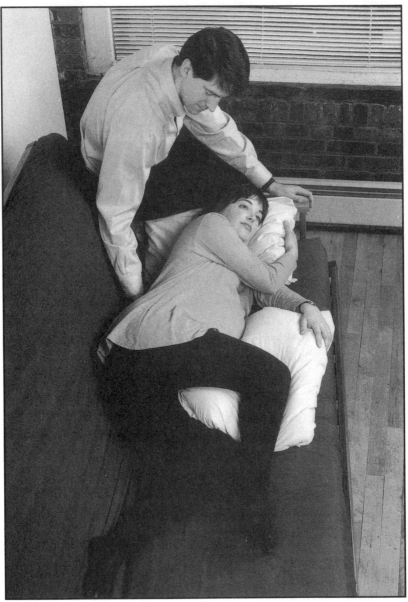

One way to alleviate discomfort in back labor is to lie on your side with partner exerting pressure on lower back.

possible to alleviate the discomfort of back labor in a number of ways:

counter pressure

change of position

change of temperature

1. Instead of massaging your abdomen, you can massage or put pressure on your back. Back labor is usually felt in two distinct points low on your back, near the sacrum.

Massaging your back is fine, but does not really help you to

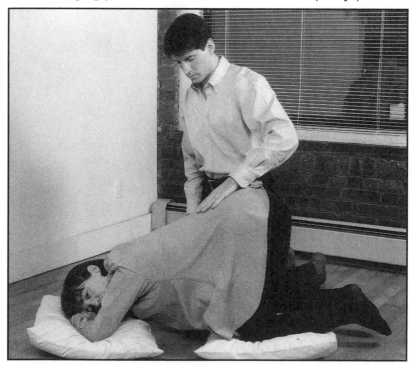

The knee-chest position for back labor

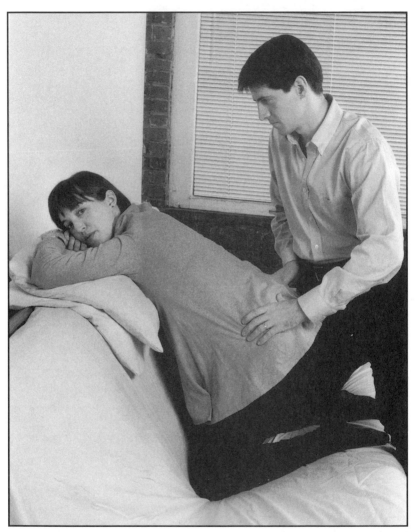

Kneeling on bed and leaning against raised head of bed is an excellent position for back labor.

relax. Your partner's help at this point will be invaluable. He can massage your back, or put counter pressure against the points that hurt during a contraction. He can put a good deal of pressure on your back and need not worry about hurting you at all. The uterus is far away from the area he will be pressing against. In fact, the more pressure he exerts against the painful areas, the better you will feel.

When your partner has been pressing his fists into your back for two hours or more, not only will his back be sore, but his knuckles will be rubbed through. We therefore suggest that you bring two tennis balls or a can of tennis balls to lean against and give your husband a rest. Actually, anything hard will do the trick. The tennis balls will also go into your Lamaze bag. They will give the counter pressure in your back and relieve some of the back pain.

Tell your partner he does not have to worry about finding the right spot to press against. You are sure to tell him in no uncertain terms to move his hand or fist to the left, to the right, to the middle, or up or down.

2.   Change your position. What would you think the aim in changing position to be? The simple answer is: Get the baby off your back! As long as you are half sitting or perhaps even lying on your back, you have the weight of the baby on your spine, which definitely aggravates back labor. You will probably find it far more comfortable to lie on your side, allowing the weight of the baby to be carried by the bed. Bend both knees, placing the upper knee in front of the lower one, and support the upper knee and your abdomen with a pillow. It is best to lie on your left side.

You may also feel perfectly comfortable sitting up at an angle of 90 degrees. Have your husband roll up your bed, but do not lean against the back of the bed. Round your back and put a pillow for support against the lower part of your spine.

Another position which some women find helpful is what we call the "knee-chest" position (page 85). You kneel and rest your body on your lower arms and hands. In this position the weight of the baby is entirely off your spine, and may provide excellent relief from all back pressure. Many women also use this position when suffering from severe menstrual cramps. A very good variation here would be to kneel on the bed and at the same time to lean against the rolled-up bed (page 86). In this position, the weight of the baby would be off your spine, gravity would help to move the baby down, and the pressure of the baby's head against the cervix might help the dilation. Try out these positions and practice the breathing exercises with them—this way you will be prepared for any changes that may occur during your labor.

You could also sit on the edge of the bed, feet resting on a chair. Use the bed table with a pillow to rest your arms and shoulders. This will be less tiring than the kneeling position.

3.   While you are still at home, during the early stages of labor, you might like to take a warm bath. The buoyancy of the water will take the weight off the uterus and help you relax. Taking a bath can only be considered if your membranes have not broken yet. If they have, a warm shower may feel good. You may find a heating pad or hot-water bottle very beneficial for back labor. I am afraid we are usually not allowed to use heating pads in the hospital.

In the hospital you could use a coolpack or Scotch ice or any of the picnic coolers that you can freeze beforehand in the freezing compartment of your refrigerator. Freezing, i.e., anesthetizing the area that hurts with a cold compress, may relieve back pain. Some hospitals offer a shower or jacuzzi where the warm water can be directed toward a painful back. Moist heat has been proven particularly helpful in alleviating the pain of back labor.

All these methods alleviate the discomfort of back labor. You will have to experiment once you are in labor and discover which method is best for you.

SECOND BREATHING TECHNIQUE

We will now discuss the second part of the first stage of labor, a period during which the cervix dilates approximately from 3 to 8 centimeters. Contractions are now becoming stronger, they last from 45 to 60 seconds, the intervals are now less than 5 minutes, most likely between 2 and 3 minutes. First-phase breathing is usually no longer effective once contractions have reached this accelerated pace. You will now need a second tool to control the strong waves. Let's say we have to shift into second gear.

Our aim must be to speed up the breathing, making it much more shallow, as if beginning a fast sprint. If one starts running, one's breathing speeds up. In this accelerated phase, the uterus works harder, and you must react to this with more rapid breathing. This allows the hard-working uterine muscle to function more efficiently and also to bring more oxygen to the uterus and to your baby.

I want to give you a few pointers before you try out this faster, shallow breathing.

Start, as always, with a deep, relaxing, cleansing breath. You can do this breathing either through your mouth or through your nose. The advantage of practicing it through your nose is that your throat and mouth will not get so dry. It is up to you, however. If you try breathing through your mouth, keep both passages open so that you will always feel a little air coming through your nose as well. This helps a great deal in relaxing the facial muscles. Breathe lightly and evenly, accentuating your exhalation slightly. You will find that the inhalation is a reflex; but you will have to concentrate on making the exhalation short and staccato, so that your breaths stay shallow and even. Breathe quietly; in fact, don't make any noise at all.

Remember to keep your neck muscles relaxed. Open your mouth very slightly, almost as if you were smiling. This will help you do this breathing almost in your throat.

Try this breathing technique very slowly at first. It may help you to beat a rhythm with your fingers. It has also helped some women to breathe in certain rhythms, stressing every first breath in four—for example, a little song in 4/4 rhythm. I've found that "Frère Jacques" gives a wonderful beat to breathe to. Be sure to make the "Frère Jacques" very "moderato." If you find yourself going "allegro vivace," you can be sure your breathing is much too fast. I'd rather have you err on the slow side than breathe too fast.

Don't be too ambitious when you first try this breathing technique. It is easy to become discouraged. Remember that it is quite difficult, and must be practiced over a long period of time. I would advise you to try it several times a day. Begin by doing it for 15 seconds only, then increase it to 30 seconds. Eventually you should be able to breathe easily and evenly for about 45 seconds to a minute without undue fatigue.

If you lose the rhythm, overexpand your chest by breathing in more air than you breathe out, or if you get tired, blow out all the air in your lungs and resume the breathing immediately. Always begin and end your practice with a cleansing breath and a smile.

SECOND BREATHING TECHNIQUE IN LABOR

Now I am going to show you how to apply this new breathing technique in labor.

Look again at the diagram showing the second part of the first stage of labor, the accelerated phase (page 92). The waves representing intensity of contraction are fairly high. You will see from the drawing that each wave increases in intensity as it rises and decreases in intensity as it subsides.

Your task at this point is to follow the wave of the contraction. There is no sense in exhausting yourself by breathing rapidly from beginning to end of the wave. Remember that one of our main objectives is to channel our energies and be as economical as possible with our muscle power.

You must therefore start the contraction with a cleansing breath and then start to breathe slowly, increasing your rate of breathing as the contraction increases in intensity. Breathe in a 4/4 rhythm at the peak of the contraction, but immediately slow down your breathing as the contraction tapers off. Conclude with another cleansing breath and a smile. In this way you will stay with the wave, accelerating when the contraction builds up and declerating as it subsides. It is as if you are running a race with the contraction, but a race in which you must only keep parallel.

I will now give you the commands for this second breathing technique. Contraction begins: focus your eyes on one point or have eye contact with your partner. Take a cleansing breath and relax your whole body. Start to breathe slowly but take shallow breaths. Now the contraction is getting stronger, stronger, stronger. It is at its peak. It is still at its peak. It is still there. It is still there, and now it begins to subside, slower and slower and slower and slower. Contraction is over. Take a deep cleansing breath and smile.

After you have practiced accelerating and decelerating your breathing for a few days, I want you to add the effleurage, or massage of your abdomen. This is difficult and needs a great deal of coordination, as the massage has to be performed slowly, regularly and lightly, as your breathing builds up and slows down.

When practicing this breathing by yourself, I want you to give exact commands in your own mind. Watch a clock with a second hand, and say to yourself, "Contraction begins!" Then slowly increase your rate of breathing so that you get to the peak within 10 to 15 seconds, stay at the peak for about 20 to 30 seconds, slow down for 15 to 20 seconds. Conclude by saying, "Contraction ends!"

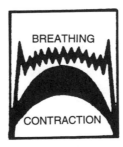

YOUR PARTNER SIMULATES A CONTRACTION

If your partner practices with you, let him put his hand just above your knee, and as he gives you the command "Contraction begins!" let him put pressure on your thigh. He should increase the pressure slowly, coming to the peak of his pressure in about 10 to 15 seconds, keeping it up for about 20 to 30 seconds, then reducing the pressure slowly for about another 15 to 20 seconds.

In this way we are simulating, in a sense, a uterine contraction. You will be reacting to an actual physical discomfort which increases in intensity, comes to a peak and decreases again. Try it. After you have tried this, ask your partner to press your leg once while you're not breathing rapidly just as hard as he did it before. I am sure you will discover that the pressure is quite a painful sensation without your breathing technique.

Practice in different positions in order to be prepared for labor and be sure to be absolutely relaxed at all times. Also remind your partner to watch you closely and correct any mistakes he sees.

THE TRANSITION

You will remember that during the transition period the cervix dilates from about 7 or 8 centimeters to 10 centimeters, or 3½ or 4 to 5 fingers. The contractions are now more severe than at any previous time. Before I tell you about the breathing for the transition period, I want to mention some symptoms that may occur during this phase of your labor.

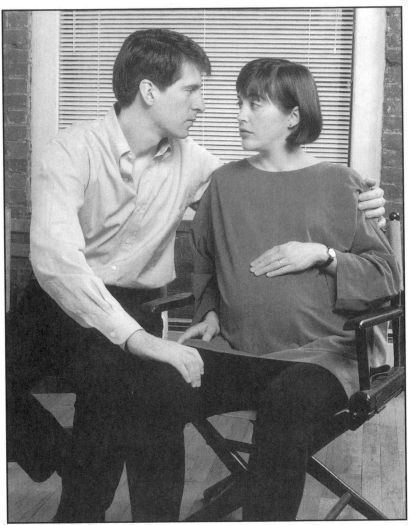

Simulating a contraction, Phil puts pressure on Sue's thigh and she follows this sensation with appropriate breathing.

1.   One of the most common symptoms at this point in labor is for the woman to become panicky. She may say: "I've had enough! Get the doctor! This is more than I bargained for! Get me out of this!" I always feel that this panic is a sure sign that you are really at the end of this first stage of labor; either you are fully dilated already, or you are 5 to 10 minutes away from it.

2.   Frequently there is a bloody, mucus discharge at this time. Nurses often call this a "good bloody show." This is caused by pressure from the baby's head against the cervix, which is extremely sensitive and has many delicate, superficial blood vessels. These little blood vessels may break. You will suddenly notice that you are getting rather wet. It is important for you and your partner to know that a "bloody show" at this point is normal. In fact it is a sign that the baby's head is descending and that you are getting closer to full dilation, and the second stage of labor.

3.   Most women will feel an increasing amount of pressure in the rectum at this point. You may also have back labor, even if up to now you have felt labor only in your lower abdomen. You may find that sitting upright and leaning slightly forward will alleviate a great deal of back pressure, or perhaps even lying on your side. Also, instead of massaging your abdomen, put your hands over your coccyx (the lowest vertebra of your spine) and press hard. Better still, let your partner press upward against your coccyx.

4.   It is possible that you will already feel a slight desire to push at this point. However, it is most important that you do not push until your physician has examined you and given explicit permission to do so. The desire to push is a reflex set off by pressure of the baby's head against the vaginal walls, the rectum and the pelvic floor. Occasionally this reflex occurs

before you are fully dilated. It is imperative, therefore, that you act against this reflex and don't push until dilation is complete. If you try to push the baby through an opening that is too small, you will have unnecessary pain, you will waste a great deal of valuable effort and you will risk a swelling of your cervix. There is a very easy way to counteract the urge to push. It can be done by forcibly exhaling, or blowing out air until the urge has passed. You know, of course, that when you try to expel a stool, you hold your breath. Even if you are lifting a heavy weight, you hold your breath to do so.

Try the following exercise: Hold your breath and strain. Now blow out continuously, always breathing in *and* out, and try to strain at the same time. Notice that this is almost impossible. You will understand now why I ask you to blow out forcibly and continually during labor whenever you get an early urge to push and have been told not to.

You cannot, of course, stop your uterus from pushing. Remember, it is an involuntary muscle. However, you can stop yourself from adding weight to the uterus. It will feel as if the lower part of your body is going in one direction and you have to keep the upper part of your body away from the lower. Don't ever think you have failed when you feel your uterus pushing downward. All you can do is to try not to add any weight to it.

5. Some women feel nauseated during transition and may even vomit. Please realize that if this should happen to you, these unpleasant symptoms are within the normal course of events. Don't be frightened if they occur.

6. Occasionally a woman will start to shake or tremble. You may find that it becomes more and more difficult to relax. You may feel hot and cold, and your control of the uterine waves may become more and more difficult.

I would like to tell you about one of my students whom I had warned about these possible unpleasant symptoms during the transition period. Apparently she had not really believed that anything like that could happen to her. But there she was in transition, her legs shaking like a leaf. She didn't become frightened, but she thought it was so funny that she started to laugh. She kept on pointing at her trembling legs and laughing. The nurse in attendance thought my student had lost her mind. She had certainly never before seen anybody laugh during the transition.

7. Finally, there is one more symptom I want to mention. Almost every woman gets terribly irritable during this phase of labor. Up to now you have been grateful for your partner's help: his rubbing your back, wetting your lips with a sponge, encouraging you. Now suddenly you may find yourself snapping at him: "Don't touch me. Don't talk to me, leave me alone!" Partners must be aware of this possibility and remember that this bad temper is only temporary. It will disappear as soon as you are fully dilated and have been given permission to push.

BREATHING DURING TRANSITION

In order to stay in control during these extremely strong contractions, we need a new breathing technique, which is even more precise and demands even more concentrated effort on our part. A stronger, more forceful rhythm has to be established. As an obstetrician once observed, "You have to become Rockettes in labor," which means that you have to work with the kind of precision the Rockettes use in Radio City Music Hall. We can do this best by using 2, 4 or 6 short breaths,

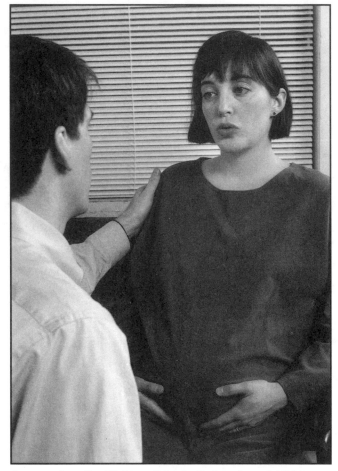

Sue practices the third breathing technique by establishing a strict pattern; 6 quick breaths followed by a short blow.

followed by a quick exhalation (through pursed lips), continuing this pattern until the end of the contraction, which may now last as long as 1-1/2 minutes.

The *short* exhalation after 2, 4 or 6 breaths should be just like a short accent. Be sure to make it quite short—don't rest on it by breathing too slowly. Do not forget to use the cleansing breath here at the beginning and end of the contraction. These strong transition contractions are likely to reach the peak of their intensity within 5 seconds of the beginning, so you will have no time to accelerate slowly. Use the very rapid breathing immediately after the cleansing breath, and only slow down when the contraction begins to taper off. Do not massage your abdomen any more during this period, but do have a specific place for your hands. Support your abdomen with them, for example, putting slight pressure on your groin. Or you may prefer pressing your hands against your coccyx.

Should you feel a desire to push during such a contraction, blow out continuously, remembering to breathe in after each forcible exhalation. Then return to the breathe-and-blow pattern, once the urge to push has subsided, for as long as the contraction continues.

I suggest that you use the transition breathing once your contractions begin to come as rapidly as 1-1/2 minutes apart, regardless of whether you experience any of the other symptoms mentioned earlier.

Remember that you must react to *your* specific uterine contractions and not to a preconceived idea of what your labor should be like. Let me repeat again: every labor is different from every other. You may experience innumerable variations of my description of labor. But the great advantage of the Lamaze technique is that it provides you with enough techniques to stay in control of your labor, however it may vary from your expectations.

I will now give the command: Contraction begins; cleansing breath; rapid breathing—inhale-exhale, inhale-exhale, inhale-short blow. Repeat: inhale-exhale, etc. (*do not blow out too much air or you may hyperventilate*) blow out, 1, 2, etc.

Contraction over, cleansing breath, smile . . . and rest. Make the most of the rest between contractions. Save energy!

Here is some advice to the coach. It happens frequently that your partner will suddenly say, "I've had enough, I'm giving up, I can't make it" or something to that effect. Go and get the nurse or doctor and ask him or her to examine your wife. The chances are she is either fully dilated or 5 to 10 minutes away from it.

The untrained woman will feel like giving up at 5- or 6-centimeter dilation. The trained woman will want to quit when she is almost ready to push her baby out.

This rapid breathing will make you thirsty, particularly if you breathe through your mouth. Many hospitals will not allow you to drink anything during labor except an occasional sip of water. You may also be offered some crushed ice. I advise you, therefore, to bring some lollipops or a peppermint stick to the hospital, so that you can lubricate your mouth a little between contractions.

You can bring a "Lamaze bag," which can, of course, be any old shopping bag, and which will hold your can of talcum powder, the lollipops or peppermint sticks, a small paper bag to breathe in, in case you hyperventilate, and some other items that you will find on the complete list on pages 129 to 132.

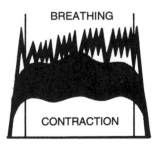

BREATHING

CONTRACTION

LESSON 5

*The second stage of labor; what happens during actual
delivery and how to prepare for it; partner's role during
delivery; how to stop pushing on command.*

We have now covered the entire first stage of labor, and you have learned the techniques that will be used during this long period. Before discussing the second stage, or *explusion*, it is imperative to review all our exercises, relaxation techniques and breathing methods.

Do you remember what to do if you have back labor? You will recall that the breathing techniques remain the same whether your labor is felt in your abdomen or your back, and that there are changes of position that will help. You should roll your bed up to an angle of 90 degrees. Do not lean back, but bend slightly forward and put a pillow against your lower back. This will help to take the weight of the baby off your spine. You may prefer instead to try lying on your side, your upper knee resting on a pillow over the lower knee and a pillow supporting your abdomen. Another technique is the knee-chest position, in which you lean forward on all fours with your lower arms resting on a pillow, or one in which you kneel on the bed, leaning your arms and trunk against the raised bed. Or sit on the edge of your bed, feet resting on a chair, and support your arms and shoulders on a table.

We have also seen how you can ease back labor by exerting pressure on your lower back with your fingers or fists. Or your partner may massage you, pressing his hands as hard as he can against the lower part of your spine. Or you can use the tennis balls you brought along in your "Lamaze bag."

If you have back labor during transition, the kneeling position, leaning against the raised bed, may be most comfortable. But in the final analysis, it will always have to be you who decides which position, counter pressure or cold application is the most comforting at the time. If there is a great deal of rectal pressure, ask your partner or the nurse to push against your coccyx. Remember that about 25 percent of women experience back labor, so it's important to be well prepared for this possibility.

Now practice the three breathing techniques for the first stage of labor. I'm sure you will notice how much you've improved in the week or two that you have been practicing. The rapid shallow breathing should be easier to perform, your rhythm should be better—and now you probably don't get too exhausted. During the stress of actual labor your breathing will come quite easily—automatically, in fact. All your practice and training will help you to coordinate your activities, channel your energy and use your body with a minimum amount of effort.

THE SECOND STAGE OF LABOR

Expulsion is really the most wonderful stage of labor. Until now you've worked hard, concentrating on riding each wave of your contractions. You've had to relax under great stress and still perform your breathing techniques. And all this has probably gone on for a good number of hours.

During the second stage you will *still* have to work tremendously hard. But now you can help your uterus in the expulsion of your baby. It is the most satisfying and exhilarating work you will ever have to do. This stage is much shorter than the long, tedious dilation of the cervix, and you know that your baby will soon be born. You will feel during this period as if you have a second wind. Although the expulsion will be just about the hardest physical work you'll ever do in your life, it will feel absolutely wonderful.

Before I explain the technique of pushing, I want you to look again at the illustration showing the expulsion of the baby, so that you will understand the workings of your uterus, how the baby is being rotated and how you can help with the expulsion—consciously, in order to expel your baby smoothly. You will be able to do this, because you have been practicing the pelvic floor exercises for many weeks.

At this point you will see again how important the Kegel exercises have been to prepare your body for the expulsion of your baby.

Once the baby is descending, there will be great pressure on your rectum. It is now imperative for you to be able to relax the pelvic floor.

WHAT HAPPENS DURING DELIVERY

Look once again at the illustrations on pages 31 and 32 and visualize how the baby is expelled from the uterus. Think also of how you can help with your own pushing to bring the baby out as smoothly and quickly as possible. You can see that as the baby enters the vagina, or birth canal, it rotates 90 degrees, and now faces the mother's spine. The baby's head bends down when it reaches the pelvic floor, so that the crown of its head shows first at the exit of the vagina, or vulva. You can see now why the doctor will talk of "the baby's head crowning."

If you are in a birthing room you will be able to labor and deliver your baby in the same room and in the same bed. This eliminates being rushed in the middle of pushing to a different room and put onto a delivery table.

If a birthing room is not available, and it is your first baby, you will start pushing in the labor room and be moved to the delivery room only when about a dime-sized area of the head is showing. At this point your husband will probably be able to tell you what color hair the baby has. To push the baby down this far may take anywhere from 10 to 30 minutes. Then—in the delivery room—the baby's head will bend back as it stretches the outlet of the vagina, and you will push it out. This should take another 15 to 20 minutes, assuming that there are no complications. If the baby is presenting posteriorly, or sunny-side up, the pushing will take much longer, and it is likely to be painful. You may also need your doctor's or midwife's help in rotating the baby's head or perhaps lifting it gently into the world with forceps. If this is your second or third or even fourth pregnancy, you will be moved into the delivery room as soon as you are fully dilated and have been given permission to push.

Now you'll need the action of the diaphragm to give additional force to the uterus in its expulsive action. You can reinforce the uterus by using your upper abdominal muscles, and by forcing down the diaphragm to help from above. Pushing the baby out is like a piston action: hard pressure from above pushing down and out. Your aim now is to reduce the intra-abdominal space and to increase the intra-abdominal pressure. This action could be best accomplished if you were allowed to assume a squatting position to expel the baby. It is interesting that about two-thirds of the women on our earth *still* give birth in the squatting position. I think we would never have to teach a woman to bear down if we could let her push the baby out while squatting. Unfortunately, modern society and modern obstetric technique demand of us that we push lying down, really against gravity and against normal instinct. Of course, it is easier for the attending physician to deal with any difficulties that may occur if the woman is lying on her back with legs raised. However, position and even designs for delivery tables are now slowly changing; that is to say, changing in such a way that the comfort of the delivering mother is considered. The Lamaze labor-delivery-bed has been accepted in a number of hospitals all over the country.

You can see how much more logical and physiologically sound this position is, and also how much more comfortable the mother is. Surely, no other mammal on this earth is asked to give birth lying flat on its back with its legs up in the air! I would recommend that you discuss giving birth in an upright position with your doctor or midwife beforehand.

But as the majority of women will still have to start their pushing in the labor room and then be moved onto a regular delivery table once a little of the head is showing, I will explain to you now how to practice the pushing in the labor bed.

Lean against your partner's legs, sitting on your tail bone at an angle of about 75 degrees from the horizontal. Rest your feet on the floor, feet and knees comfortably separated. Hold on to your knees or under your knees. Keep your elbows well out and

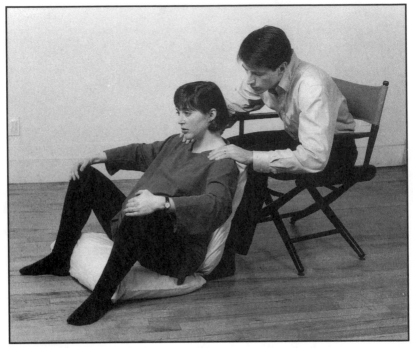

Sue and Phil practice the labor room pushing with Sue's back at about a 75° angle.

push your head forward. Your back should be rounded as it is resting against your partner's legs.

It is important that you push correctly and in a disciplined fashion so that you can expel the baby in as short a period as possible. You will have to push only with contractions and only when you have been given the okay for pushing by someone in authority, i.e., a nurse, a resident or your doctor.

The contractions will slow down somewhat when you start to push. They will probably not be as violent as your transition contractions. Don't rush into pushing. You will be more effective if you do it slowly and deliberately. Now, let us assume a contraction begins. As usual, we start by taking a deep cleansing breath. However, to get the most out of a contraction, let it build up strength first before you help the uterus in its expulsion effort. Therefore, take a second cleansing breath. Then inhale a third time deeply, let out a little of your breath, hold the remaining air, relax your lower jaw and push steadily, directing all your force through your vagina. Remember, elbows out, head forward, pelvic floor muscles relaxed. Sustain the pushing effort for about 10 seconds, let the air out, lower your head, quickly take another breath, exhale a little, hold the rest and bear down, relax your lower jaw, hold and push for 10 seconds, breathe out and let your head relax. Quickly take a third breath, exhale a little, hold the rest, relax your lower jaw, and push smoothly for 10 seconds, thinking in the direction of your vagina. Finally breathe out, and take several cleansing breaths to make up for the oxygen you didn't bring to the baby while you were pushing. It is important to remember not to hold your breath in your throat. If you do, you will strain your face and neck and waste a great deal of energy. By exhaling part of your breath and holding it at the level of your diaphragm, by keeping your mouth slightly open to prevent holding your breath in your throat, you will be able to direct the pushing effort downward. It may be helpful to count up to eight while you are pushing. Thus, you will be exhaling a little air as you push and prevent any strain in your neck and face. You could also say to yourself, "Out baby, out baby. . . ." as you are pushing. The words "Out baby" will help you to push correctly.

You can practice the pushing exercise safely every day, holding your breath for 6 to 10 seconds. During actual labor, however, you will have to sustain your pushing efforts for a longer period. Usually you'll need three breaths and three pushes for one contraction. And in actual labor you will reinforce your uterus with deliberate muscular efforts. Each time you push, the baby will descend a certain distance, and each time the contraction is over the baby will slip back a little. It's really like taking two steps forward and one back. Therefore, the more you can relax your pelvic floor muscles, the faster your baby will be born.

PARTNER'S ROLE DURING EXPULSION

Your partner can be of great assistance in practicing this technique. He can make sure you are in a correct position. He can support your back. He can practice with you and give the pushing commands: "Breathe in—breathe out, breathe in—breathe out, breathe in—let out a little air—count to eight, allowing a little air to escape as you push, hold on to your knees, keep your elbows out and push, push, push . . . breathe out—take a second breath, let out a little, count to eight, relax your lower jaw and push . . . push . . . breathe out, quickly once more: breathe in, let out a little—hold, relax your lower lip and push, push . . . breathe out and relax."

I have found that even the best-trained woman may forget how to push. The doctor gives her the permission to push with the next contraction, and she will suddenly look up in utter panic and say: "I've forgotten how!" It is unlikely that both of you will forget the same things at the same time, and it will help you enormously if your partner can give you exact commands. You'll have to tell him when the contraction begins, and he will then give you the signals when to breathe and push. I am sure that once he has done this for two or three contractions, you'll be able to function perfectly well on your own.

Try not to be too much of a perfectionist in labor. It may take you a few contractions until you really feel that you are pushing well. Don't be discouraged. You will fall into the correct pattern of pushing very quickly, particularly if you and your partner have trained together and are allowed to work together during labor and delivery.

THE DELIVERY-ROOM TABLE

In case you cannot use a birthing bed, I want to describe pushing on a delivery table. The pushing technique that you will use on the delivery table is the same that you used in the labor room. The delivery-room table is very much like the table in your doctor's office: hard, flat and narrow. But instead of putting your heels into stirrups, as you do in your doctor's office, your legs will be supported under your knees and thighs. This is much more comfortable. Unfortunately, in most hospitals the delivery table cannot be raised so that you can push down from above. You should therefore bring your pillows from the labor room into the delivery room to support your shoulders and head. A few hospitals may provide a backrest on the delivery table or a foam-rubber bolster.

You will have handles or grips to hold onto, or you may hold the vertical bars that attach the stirrups to the table. These handles or bars will enable you to pull yourself up when you have to push.

In order to allow for the most comfortable position to push, ask that the stirrups be lowered, so that you can raise your back to an angle of about 40 to 45 degrees. If the table cannot be raised, or if there is no backrest available, push the pillows you've brought from the labor room well under your back, not just under your head and shoulders.

It is of great advantage to practice pushing in the actual positions you're likely to use during real labor. In this way, you can train your body and muscles to function well in the proper positions from the very beginning.

When you are on the delivery table your legs and your abdomen will be draped with sterile material. Be sure never to touch the sterile drapes! Keep your hands firmly on the bars. It used to be common to strap a woman's wrists in order to make sure that she would not inadvertently touch the sterile drapes placed over her abdomen and legs. However, this medieval custom has been discontinued in all hospitals. Everyone knows that a trained woman will not touch any drapes or sheets she has been asked not to touch. It will be difficult for you to watch the emergence of your child, because you are too low and the drape obstructs your view. But frequently there is a mirror above the delivery table, which can be easily adjusted so that you can watch your baby being born. Occasionally it may be easier to push your baby out in a different position. This may be especially so if you've had back labor, i.e., if your baby presented posteriorly or sunny-side up. Pushing in the "Sims" position, which is on your side, will encourage the baby to turn anteriorly, make the pushing easier for you and come out faster. To take up this position, you lie on your left side, bend both knees and hold your right leg under your thigh. Your partner could also support the upper leg for you. You will then use the same pushing technique as before: Two cleansing breaths to let the contraction build up, then inhale deeply, let out half the air, keep your mouth slightly open and relaxed, hold the residual air with your diaphragm (make sure not to hold your breath in

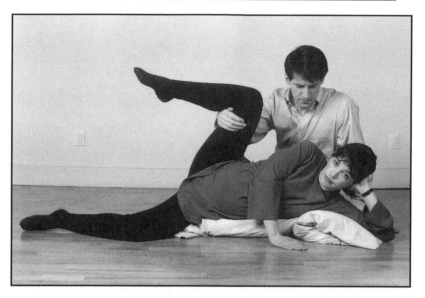

Side-lying position for pushing.

your throat) and push. Repeat this until the contraction is over. You probably need 3 to 4 breaths or pushes for one contraction.

Another alternative is to squat in order to facilitate the rotation of the baby's head. You can squat in bed, holding on to your husband or coach. Sometimes you may be told to start pushing on a commode or toilet to encourage the descent of the baby. Modern birthing beds have a metal bar you can hold on to while you squat to push the baby out.

HOW TO STOP PUSHING ON COMMAND

At the moment your baby's head emerges and begins rotating to allow the shoulders to come out, your doctor may tell you to stop pushing. It is of the utmost importance that you are

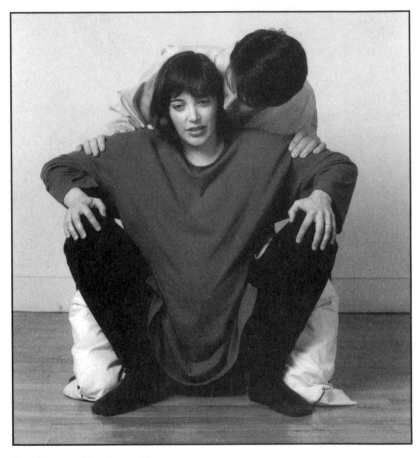

Squatting position for pushing.

prepared to cooperate immediately. Lean back, relax your body and blow out repeatedly until the urge to push is over. In a short time your doctor will advise you to continue pushing, but this pause is likely to be a difficult moment for you. The urge to push will probably be extremely strong and you will be asked to counteract this strong involuntary feeling. It's quite possible to prepare for this moment if, in your expulsion exercises at home, you let your husband occasionally give you the command "stop pushing," and you learn to react instantaneously.

DAILY EXERCISE REVIEW

NEUROMUSCULAR CONTROL EXERCISES
(see Lesson Two)

Sit comfortably in a chair, your arms and feet well supported.

1. Contract right arm. Release.
2. Contract right leg. Release.
3. Contract right arm, right leg. Release.
4. Contract right arm, left leg. Release.

Repeat with left arm and left leg. Always be sure to relax the rest of the body when contracting arms and legs. Practice daily, coach giving commands and checking relaxation.

STRETCHING EXERCISES
(see Lesson Two)

Practice every day on a hard surface (not in bed) without pillows.

1. Sit cross-legged (tailor fashion) on the floor, back relaxed and slightly rounded. Use this position as much as possible.

2.   Sit on the floor. Put the soles of your feet together, then pull feet as near your body as possible. Press knees gently toward floor. Repeat three to five times.

3.   Pelvic rocking: On all fours: Inhale, then exhale—tuck your tail in and lower your head—inhale and straighten your head and back. Repeat ten times.

4.   Lie on back with legs bent, knees and feet separated, feet firmly on the floor. Inhale through nose and raise back off the floor, pushing hips toward the ceiling. Exhale slowly through mouth and lower back bit by bit, keeping hips up till the end. Relax. Repeat three times.

5.   Sit cross-legged, stretch arms overhead and look up. Stretch more. Stretch more. Repeat three to five times.

BREATHING EXERCISES
(see Lessons Three and Four)

1.   Preliminary labor (30 to 45 second contractions): Eye contact with coach or focal point. Cleansing breath. Slow, rhythmic chest breathing, inhaling through nose, exhaling through lips, 6 to 9 breaths per minute. Cleansing breath and smile. Practice with massage (effleurage) for abdomen or back. One minute, three times daily.

2.   Accelerated or Active Labor (45 to 60 second contractions): Eye contact with coach or focal point. Cleansing breath. Slow, shallow breaths through either mouth or nose, accelerating as contraction builds, decelerating as contraction subsides. Cleansing breath and smile. Practice with effleurage, one minute, three times daily.

3.   Transition (60 to 90 second contractions): Eye contact with coach or focal point. Support abdomen with both hands from below. Cleansing breath. Pattern of 2, 4 or 6 shallow, short breaths, followed by one light, short blow. Repeat until contraction is over. Cleansing breath and smile. Practice for 60 to 90 seconds, three times daily. Also practice blowing out to avoid pushing.

EXPULSION EXERCISES
(see Lesson Five)

1. Kegel exercise: Contract urethra, vagina and anal sphincter. Hold to count of 3. Release. Repeat 20 to 30 times daily.
2. Pushing for labor room: Sit at a 75° angle, feet on floor, knees bent. Hold knees, elbows out, inhale, exhale. Inhale, exhale. Inhale, exhale a little, relax lower lip and push, counting to eight with each push. Sustain for a count of eight. Exhale. Inhale quickly, exhale a little, hold breath, relax lower lip and push. Sustain for a count of eight. Exhale. Inhale quickly, exhale a little, hold breath, relax lower lip and push. Exhale. Relax. Several cleansing breaths and smile. Practice once daily.

LESSON 6

Recognizing real labor; what to bring along; moment-to-moment at the hospital; breathing with your labor; use of medication; the great moment and after.

I'm sure you have often wondered: How will I know when my labor begins? How will I be able to tell the difference between the kind of contractions I've been having for the last few weeks and the real ones? I've heard that perhaps I can sleep through part of my labor—is this true?

These are very legitimate questions. One good basic rule to follow is this: when you feel slight contractions and you are not sure whether this is real labor or not, the chances are it is *not*. Yes, you can sleep through early labor, but any contraction that doesn't wake you is obviously so mild that you don't have to concentrate on it. I have often found that the doctor and the laboring mother do not agree on when labor started. For the woman, it feels like labor when the contractions are obvious enough for her to be aware of them. They may be mild, but she is excited, she knows she should not eat any more, and she listens carefully to every little sign and symptom her body gives her. Finally she wants to know for certain and calls the doctor, who may tell her to come to the hospital to be examined. She arrives at the hospital and is examined, and the doctor tells her that she is not in labor yet.

This is very upsetting. She has been having contractions for hours by now, she has not eaten anything, she has been awake most of the night, and now the doctor tells her that this is not labor yet. What are those contractions, and when will they become effective so that the cervix begins to dilate? she asks herself. She is already tired, and the doctor tells her she has not even started labor yet. This can be a difficult time.

There are, however, certain definite indications that you should be aware of. Therefore I would like to discuss with you now the signs with which we associate the beginning of labor.

1. You may observe an increase in mucus discharge toward the end of your pregnancy. At one point this discharge will probably be tinged with a little blood. This will indicate the expulsion of the mucous plug which closes the cervix during your pregnancy. It is generally just a very slight stain, which you will notice only when you go to the bathroom. If no other symptoms—such as contractions or breaking of the membrane—occur simultaneously, don't get too excited at this point. It may be hours or even days before you will go into real labor. Therefore, losing the mucous plug is not necessarily a reliable indication of the beginning of labor.

2. The second indication of the beginning of labor is the onset of actual contractions. Contractions do not always start as the textbooks tell us: first about 20 minutes apart, gradually getting closer together and becoming more regular. It is just as normal for the contractions to begin only 5 minutes apart. Do not become alarmed if this occurs. It is a perfectly normal variation. It *is* important that you keep track of the intensity of the contractions, noting whether they last 30 seconds or more and if the intervals between them become shorter.

Although the uterine muscle is an involuntary muscle—like your heart or stomach—it is affected by your emotions. Just as you feel your heart beating violently if you are frightened or upset, or your stomach "turning over" if you are very nervous, so your uterus also reacts to anxieties. If you become very excited and tense, it may contract repeatedly—but, unfortunately, with no results. Therefore, your understanding of the process of labor will help you immensely in approaching your delivery. You can avoid unnecessary tension and allow your body to work smoothly during your labor. This understanding and knowledge will also help you give the doctor or midwife an accurate description of what's happening when you contact him/her at the onset of labor. Your physician will always give you exact instructions as to when he/she wants to be called and when he/she wants you to leave for the hospital.

BREAKING OF WATER

Breaking of water, or rupturing the membranes that contain the amniotic fluid in which the baby lives during your pregnancy, may occur at any time during your labor. You may become aware of a slow leaking or feel a sudden gush of fluid. This amniotic fluid is transparent and is therefore easily distinguishable from urine. You may have noticed, toward the end of your pregnancy, that you occasionally have difficulty in controlling your urine. A sudden sneeze, a laugh or cough can make it difficult for you to hold back the urine. But you *can* control it, whereas if your membranes leak, you cannot stop the escaping fluid by contracting your muscles. This will be a positive indication that the fluid you are losing is amniotic fluid and not urine. (Since your membranes may break while you are in bed, it's a good idea to put a rubber or plastic sheet on your mattress about a week before your due date.)

I'm sure your doctor will have given you instructions to call him/her as soon as your membranes break. It is generally felt that the baby should be born within 24 to 36 hours after the membranes have broken. Your doctor or midwife will give you instructions as to when to come to the hospital. Contractions may not start spontaneously with the breaking of the waters. Your doctor will therefore ask you to come to the hospital after a few hours, so that he/she can start your labor with a hormone called Pitocin. This is given intravenously and will generally cause contractions to come hard and fast. Stronger and faster, in fact, than if your labor progressed by itself (or, as I like to call it, "organically"). So be prepared to be alert and on your toes if your labor has to be induced. I am sure you can manage it. The important thing is to know that Pitocin is likely to increase the intensity of the contractions considerably, so that you are physically and mentally prepared for this kind of labor.

Let me assure you that breaking of the membranes is entirely painless and that there is no definite time when you will lose this amniotic fluid. It's even possible that your physician will have to break the bag of waters artificially during your labor.

If your membranes break early in labor, it does not mean that you will have a "dry labor." Actually the fluid that you lose at the beginning of labor is only the tiny amount between the widest diameter of the baby's head and the cervix. Most of the fluid will be plugged off by the baby's head and shoulders. Don't worry if additional water escapes from time to time, especially during a contraction. The uterus keeps making more water, so there will be plenty left for the baby to remain cushioned and to help it finally emerge. Generally, the amniotic fluid is like water, transparent, with no particular smell. Occasionally, however, you might notice that the fluid is discolored, slightly brownish or greenish. If this is the case, tell your doctor or midwife immediately. The reason for this discoloration is that some of the baby's waste products may have been squeezed into the surrounding amniotic fluid. This waste material is a blackish, tarry mass called meconium. Your doctor or midwife will want to take precautions by watching you and the baby carefully if the fluid is dark. I am mentioning it here because it is something you can diagnose yourself easily and report to your doctor or midwife.

WHAT TO DO WHEN CONTRACTIONS BEGIN

If contractions start at night and are mild and far apart, try to rest as much as possible. Sleep between contractions as much as you can, so that you are well rested when your labor becomes more active and demands undivided attention. You can be sure that strong, advanced contractions will keep you awake, so make the most of your rest and ignore the beginning of labor as long as you can.

It may be impossible to sleep, however. That's very understandable, too. After all, you have been waiting anxiously for this moment for a long time. But I suggest that you do not lie awake in the dark. Get out of bed and take a comfortable bath in relaxing warm water, or if your membranes have broken, take a shower. Then go to the kitchen and make yourself some tea and drink it with lots of sugar or honey. The tea is a stimulant and the sugar is energy-giving. If, after all this activity, you find that labor is progressing—the contractions are increasing in frequency and intensity—you will have to be up anyhow. If, on the other hand, your contractions have slowed down again and there seems to be little change in their character, go back to bed and sleep. You'll probably be very tired in the middle of the night, and sleep may come fairly easily once you have reassured yourself that you can be in control of the situation. Don't wake your husband until you need his help and support. He will better be able to do his part if he is well rested, too.

If labor starts during the day, cut down your intake of food and fluids.

May I suggest that you prepare some Jell-O a few days before your due date and keep it in the refrigerator. Jell-O is an ideal snack early in labor. Should you become hungry, broth and light food such as fruit or crackers or yogurt or sherbet will also help you if the beginning of labor is long. Do not drink any more milk. Remember that milk is a whole food and that it is hard to digest once labor has started.

Once labor has started in earnest your digestive system automatically stops working. Anything you eat remains undigested in the stomach. I am sure you have noticed even now, during your pregnancy, how distressed you can feel after a meal. There simply is not enough space any more. You can imagine how much more uncomfortable it will be if your stomach stops working. A full stomach may cause vomiting during labor. And should you for any reason require an inhalation anesthetic, it will be infinitely easier to have it on an empty stomach.

I'd like to suggest here that for about one to two weeks before your due date, you have your last meal of the day no later than 7:30 or 8:00 P.M.—and avoid midnight snacks.

Do not immediately lie down when labor begins. If you had a good night's rest go on with your regular activities without tiring yourself. Call your husband home, if he has already left for work. It will be much nicer for you to have him there than to wonder whether he can make it back in time to take you to the hospital.

Then go for a walk, go to the movies, or visit friends, but don't tell them that you are in early labor. They might get too excited. Or start celebrating the baby's birthday by having a drink. Liquor or wine will help to determine whether this is labor proper or not, because alcohol will calm the uterus if it's only practicing. One drink is enough. If you are in false or very early labor, it will soothe the uterine muscle and contractions will slow down. If it is real labor, all it will do is make you feel a little relaxed. If you don't drink, simply vary your activities (walk if you've been sitting for a while), watch what your body is doing and follow your doctor's advice about when you should come to the hospital.

Do *not* start any deliberate breathing during contractions until you absolutely feel the need for it. As long as you can walk or talk through a contraction, there is no need to use any specific breathing technique. You'll probably feel a strong temptation to start the deliberate breathing too early, out of pure enthusiasm and excitement that you are at long last in labor. But labor will seem endless if you start controlling it before there is any actual need. You'll tire yourself needlessly, wasting valuable energy that you'll need once labor progresses and the contractions demand concentrated control. Always remember that you must channel your energies, and that from the beginning to the end of your labor you will use the techniques that you have learned, deliberately and with considerable self-discipline.

VISIT TO THE HOSPITAL AND
WHAT TO TAKE TO THE HOSPITAL

It is always a good idea to visit your hospital or birthing center well beforehand, if only to find out a good way to get there, where the night entrance and the admitting office are located, and to see the labor rooms, the delivery room, the nursery and the room you will stay in after you have the baby. Many hospitals have organized tours for expectant parents. Ask your doctor or midwife for information, or call the hospital's obstetric department.

Don't be upset if you are told of hospital procedures that you had not anticipated. Your doctor frequently has his or her own way of conducting labors, which may vary from hospital routine. Should you still have questions after the tour, don't hesitate to discuss them with your doctor or midwife.

Pack your suitcase at least two weeks before your due date. If you're going to nurse the baby, pack two nursing bras. Be sure that you do not buy nursing bras that come with a protective pad. These pads are usually made of some kind of plastic and do not allow for ventilation. The hospital will provide you with gauze pads for protection. (You can buy boxes of these pads at any drugstore, but you might find it cheaper to use old handkerchiefs or cut up an old sheet once you're home again.) Put two or three shorty nightgowns, a robe and slippers into your suitcase and, if you plan to nurse, be sure that the nightgowns open in front. This will enable you to nurse your baby without having to slip out of your nightgown at each feeding. The hospital will provide you with sanitary napkins. Do not use tampons until you've had your postpartum examination and your doctor has given you permission. Have a separate bag ready for clothes and diapers for the baby. Put out the clothes you want to wear going home, so your husband won't have a last-minute search through closets and drawers. And don't expect to fit into your tightest skirts or dresses right away.

CONTENTS OF THE LAMAZE BAG

Do you remember the Lamaze bag I told you to take to the hospital? Here is the list of things to put into your Lamaze bag:

1. Some food for your partner or coach. This is especially useful if you happen to labor at night. Few hospitals have food at nighttime, and your partner will get ravenously hungry, because he is working every moment of your labor with you. Luckily, you yourself will not be hungry during labor; also, you won't be allowed to eat. But once you've given birth, you will probably be very hungry. So tell your partner to save a sandwich for you.

2. Some lollipops or peppermint sticks to suck on between contractions if you find that your mouth has become dry from the rapid superficial breathing. Generally you will not be allowed to drink water during labor, though you might be given a little crushed ice or be allowed to rinse your mouth. A lollipop or peppermint stick will feel good and even give you a little sugar.

3.   A washcloth or a small sponge. Your husband can wet the washcloth or sponge and refresh your face. He can even let you suck on the wet sponge a little when your mouth gets dry.

4.   A chapstick. Your lips may become very dry in labor, and your lipstick is usually not greasy enough to keep them well lubricated. A chapstick will feel good and also stay on longer than lipstick.

5.   A small paper bag to breathe in, in case you hyperventilate.

6.   A small can of talcum powder or lotion to smooth the skin when you or your partner massages your abdomen or any other part of your body.

7.   Tennis balls or a can of tennis balls for counter pressure, should you have back labor. You could even use a rolling pin.

8.   Cool pack to freeze the lower back, also in case you have back labor.

9.   Mouth spray or some lemon to freshen the breath.

10.   Heavy socks, like the warm-up socks that dancers use. You will find your feet get very, very cold and clammy in labor, as all the circulation goes to your pelvic area.

11.   Anything else you feel like putting in for practical reasons, such as a picture to focus on, or for fun, a "security blanket."

Do not put this Lamaze bag into your suitcase. Your suitcase will probably be taken immediately to the room that you will occupy once you have given birth. Carry it separately or let your husband bring it to you once he comes to the labor room.

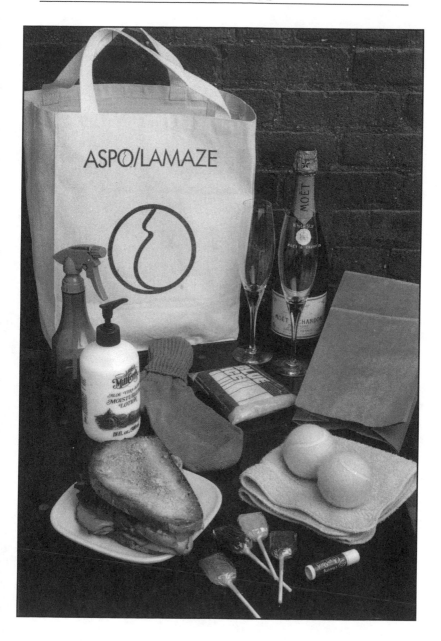

Some couples also like to include a bottle of champagne or wine to celebrate with doctors and nurses after you've given birth. Also bring some plastic glasses, for there are never enough in the hospital. Ask the nurse to put the champagne on ice when you arrive at the hospital, so it will be nice and cool when you need it.

ARRIVING AT THE HOSPITAL

When you arrive at the hospital, you will usually have to go first to the admitting office. In some hospitals your partner can attend to the registration or you can even register weeks before you actually enter the hospital. Be sure to bring any necessary insurance cards along and perhaps your checkbook. Some hospitals ask for a deposit when you arrive if you haven't given them one at early registration. Of course they will always admit you, even if you've forgotten to bring a check, but it will cause less trouble at the time if you have it along.

Should you have a contraction while signing forms, don't hesitate to let the clerk wait until you have been able to control it with the appropriate breathing techniques and it has ended. Don't feel embarrassed when stopping in the middle of signing your name. After all, you are the one who is in labor at the moment, not the person who sits behind the desk!

Make sure beforehand that your partner can stay with you when you are first taken into the labor room. It used to be that you were more or less immediately separated once you entered the hospital, and reunited only after all examinations and "prepping" had been done. Some hospitals may still try to separate you the moment you enter. Be sure to discuss this beforehand with your doctor so you don't have to start arguments or discussions in labor. I think most hospital authorities these days have come to realize that entering a hospital in labor is the first real crisis you have had to cope with. Any hospital stay is anxiety producing. But if your partner can stay with you, you will feel comforted and happy, not only to have him with you later in labor, but also at the beginning when you are being checked, examined and settled into the labor room.

You will undress completely and put on a hospital gown, a shorty that fastens in the back. This is not attractive but is quite practical. The nurse will ask you to give her a urine specimen, and she will take your temperature and your blood pressure. Then either your own doctor or a resident doctor will come and examine you. He/she will listen to the fetal heart, and check your heart and lungs. He/she will also ask you when your labor started, whether your membranes have broken, when you ate last, what you ate, etc. In many hospitals a nurse will take a blood sample to re-check your blood type, even though your doctor has done this previously at one of your prenatal visits. The doctor will then examine you internally, either rectally or vaginally. During this examination you should lie flat on your back, breathing deeply with your mouth open. This first internal examination is really most important for you. It will be the first signpost on your journey to the baby's birth. You will probably have been in labor at home for some hours, and no doubt will be eager to find out how much progress you've made so far. Your doctor may examine you during or between contractions. Be sure to ask the doctor how far you have effaced and dilated. Your own doctor will always communicate your progress to you, but don't be surprised if a resident physician seems reluctant to tell you this information. He/she doesn't know you personally and may not be aware that you are so well prepared for labor and delivery.

After this examination, a nurse will come and "prep" you. Many hospitals have changed this procedure, however. They only clip the pubic hair and shave the anal hair. In some hospitals, neither "prep" nor enema are given anymore. You should tell your doctor beforehand that you prefer this kind of partial prepping, or no prepping at all.

It's a good idea to tell the nurse, before she starts to look after you, that you are going to use the Lamaze method. Be sure to ask her not to interrupt while you are using the breathing techniques, but explain that you will be glad to answer any questions as soon as the contraction is over. You will find the nurses most cooperative and helpful. They are usually fascinated at your being able to stay in control so efficiently.

The nurse will also give you an enema if the doctor has ordered one. Frequently, women have very loose bowel movements in early labor. Should this be the case, be sure to inform your doctor or midwife so that you will not be given an enema in the hospital. Enemas are difficult enough to cope with at the best of times, and if they can be avoided in labor, it will help you to be more comfortable. If, however, you have been constipated just before labor started, or in early labor, it will feel good to have an enema, as it will give you more space. During the enema, breathe deeply through your mouth. In many hospitals you will be allowed to expel the enema on a toilet. In others you will be given a bedpan. Should you have to expel the enema on a bedpan, ask the nurse to place it on the edge of the bed and put a chair under the bed so that you can rest your feet and sit upright. Hospital beds are high and it is easy to place a chair under the bed. It is far more comfortable to expel in this way rather than having the pan placed in the middle of your bed. Stay on the toilet or bedpan for at least 20 minutes. If you don't give yourself enough time, you may find that with any subsequent contraction you will lose more stool and have to ask for another bedpan. Do not let anybody hurry you and continue with your breathing techniques whenever you have a contraction.

Ask the nurse to call your partner if he has stepped out while you had an enema. (If you know beforehand that your partner cannot stay with you during this preliminary period, tell him ahead of time that the waiting period while you are being examined and "prepped" may be from 45 minutes to one hour. This is important for him to know, since an hour may seem a very long time to him. He may worry unduly or be afraid that he has been forgotten.)

Again, remind your partner to bring a sandwich or some cookies to eat in the hospital. He may get very hungry during your labor and it may be at night when all the coffee shops are closed. Or he may feel that he does not want to leave you alone to get a snack, even for half an hour. Alas, no matter how hungry you may feel, no eating is permitted during labor!

Ask the nurse to roll your bed up to any angle that suits you. You will have to experiment a little. Don't hesitate to ask for another pillow should you need it. If you've brought your own pillows, you can use them now to make yourself more relaxed. Most women feel far more comfortable in an upright position. The breathing is easier this way, and psychologically you will feel far more in control of the situation. The only time you'll have to lie down is when the doctor examines you, or if he feels that a certain position will be better for your labor.

BREATHING WITH YOUR LABOR

Remember that no labor will follow an exact textbook pattern. There is simply no way to plan in advance what breathing you will use at any given time. The great advantage of the Lamaze method is that you have acquired techniques to use as your labor demands from moment to moment. Do not anticipate a strict pattern, but react to the sensations that you feel at the time. Every labor is different from all others; it is up to you to adjust to your labor as it occurs. However, here are some fundamental rules to keep in mind:

1. Do not start any controlled breathing until you feel the absolute need for it.

2. . Stay with the slow chest breathing as long as you can. It's much less fatiguing than the shallow, rapid breathing.

3. If you feel contractions in your back, ask your partner or the nurse to put pressure on your lower spine. You can massage or put pressure on yourself if necessary. Change positions to alleviate the discomfort of back labor by:

a. Sitting upright, leaning slightly forward so that the weight of the baby falls forward.

b. Lying on your side, placing the upper knee in front of the lower one. Place a pillow under the upper knee and abdomen so that there is no strain on your thigh muscles.

c. Using the knee-chest position to take the pressure off your back.

d. Kneeling and leaning against the raised head of the bed.

4. Ask your partner to help you stay well relaxed. He must remind you to release your arms, legs, shoulders or face whenever they get tense. You'll find that your homework pays off well here and that you will obey his commands automatically. This will give you both a feeling of doing a difficult job together.

5. Ask your partner to time the contractions and call out the intervals, 15 . . . 30 . . . 45 seconds. This will define and circumscribe the contractions. Once he calls out 45 seconds, you will know that the contraction will not go on much longer. Your beginning cleansing breath will be your husband's cue that the contraction has started. Occasionally it will be difficult for you to know exactly when the contraction has started. Your partner can help you in this case by putting his hand on the fundus, at the top of your uterus. He will usually be able to feel the tightening of the uterus with his fingers before you feel the actual sensation. He can then call out, "Now!" and you can follow this command with your cleansing breath and breathing technique. Your partner should encourage and praise you, watching to see that you perform well. We all need encouragement, love and support during labor, especially when we are awake and actively participating in childbirth.

THE FETAL MONITOR

Frequently a fetal monitor is used either externally or internally on you almost as soon as you enter the hospital. This machine monitors the fetal heartbeat, even during contractions, and at the same time shows the intensity of the uterine contractions on a paper on which a pen shows the curve pattern of the contraction. The external monitor is attached to your abdomen by two wide, elastic stockinette belts. This may make effleurage difficult, though you could confine the massage to the lower abdomen, where it is probably most beneficial anyway. The internal monitor will be attached by means of a small electrode to the presenting part of the baby, once the membranes have ruptured.

I would like to include a few words about the fetal monitor here. It is an electronic machine which is meant to assure a great safety factor for the baby during labor, as it points into the directions the staff should look if fetal heart irregularities occur. The machine is invaluable for high-risk mothers or babies. If it is used, even though you may not be a high-risk mother, use it as an added indicator—almost like using biofeedback—to recognize the beginning, strength and end of a contraction. This makes it possible to stay with contractions, catch them on time with breathing techniques, in short, ride the waves. You will be able to watch a paper emerge from the monitor and follow the pen that is drawing the exact curve of your uterine contraction. In fact, you will find that the machine registers your contractions before you are actually aware of them.

By discussing the use of the fetal monitor beforehand with your doctor or midwife, you may find that the use of the machine could be optional if your labor develops smoothly, or that the monitor could be used only from time to time to verify what every experienced physician and nurse is able to diagnose by listening to the fetal heart and using their excellent clinical experience. Machines frequently go out of order and may not be as reliable as the human ear. Also, being fastened to a machine tends to immobilize you, while it is generally felt that changing positions and moving around—or even walking—during labor can encourage uterine contractions.

It's important that you urinate whenever necessary during the first stage of labor. A large accumulation of urine may become quite uncomfortable and a full bladder takes up precious space in the abdominal cavity. You may find it a little difficult to urinate if the bladder is too full or if the uterus presses on it more and more as the baby descends. If you've had no medication, your husband can help you to the bathroom. If, however, you have had some sedation, ask the nurse for a bedpan. You may also have to use a bedpan if you are attached to a fetal monitor or if you have an intravenous drip in your wrist or lower arm.

Your doctor or midwife will examine you periodically during labor to determine what progress has been made. Always remember to ask them about your progress after each examination. If you are told how many centimeters you are dilated, it will give you a rough idea of how far along you've come. From time to time a nurse will listen to the fetal heart or watch the fetal monitor and take your blood pressure. This listening is important, as it is the only way the doctor and nurse can keep in touch with your baby during labor, and be sure that all is well.

THE USE OF MEDICATION

If at any time you should feel the need for medication or sedation, don't hesitate to ask for it. Your doctor will be happy to give you as much relief as he/she considers medically safe. If he/she suggests medication there are undoubtedly good reasons for this decision, and I am sure they will be explained and discussed with you.

You've had many months during your prenatal visits to the doctor to discuss your and your partner's active participation in the birth of your child. Any medication you may be given will be necessary to insure both the health of your baby and your own safety. There are two kinds of medication that are generally used these days:

1. Analgesics
2. Anesthetics

Analgesics: the most commonly used is Demerol, which is a synthetic in the morphine family. It is administered intravenously, and it can only be given in the first stage of labor and generally not until the cervix has dilated to 5 centimeters. It is also not recommended late in the first stage of labor, as the baby would be born too soon after the administration of the drug, and it would therefore have a more difficult time in metabolizing the drug. Demerol is often given in conjunction with a tranquilizer, Phenergan, which enhances the action of Demerol. This means that less Demerol can be given with the same effect.

As a depressant, Demerol does not take much pain away, but it does help you relax between contractions. The effect on the baby is similar to the one on you, and the drug is therefore given with great caution and in comparatively small dosages.

Anesthetics: The medication of choice these days is a regional anesthetic given into the epidural space of your spine. It has the ability to anesthetize the sensory nerves from your hips to your toes without affecting your consciousness. You will be awake and you will be able to hold your baby immediately after birth.

One of the disadvantages, however, is that it may make it more difficult for you to push the baby out. Normally we need a resistance for pushing; otherwise it would be like pushing feathers. If you have no sensation from your hips down, you may need help with the expulsion of the baby. The help could be fundal pressure, that is to say that someone presses on your abdomen to help move the baby down, or your doctor may decide to discontinue the epidural just before you are fully dilated so that you can actively help in the expulsion of your baby. Another drawback of the epidural anesthesia may be that the mother's blood pressure may suddenly drop. This can, of course, be counteracted immediately, but it may be better not to have it happen at all. One of the precautions to prevent this sudden drop in blood pressure is to give the mother an IV with glucose.

CESAREAN SECTIONS

In the case of a complicated or lengthy labor, it is frequently felt that delivery by cesarean section will benefit the baby. The decision will have to be made by your doctor, but he/she will always discuss his/her views and your options beforehand. Generally you will be given a regional anesthetic, and in most hospitals your partner can be with you during the birth if he so wishes. His role is to comfort you and talk to you during this procedure. He can talk to you, encourage you and in the end bond with you and the baby.

Most cesarean sections are not emergency operations. They are done after a thorough exploration of the benefits and risks. The most frequent reasons for a section are:

1. No progress in labor.
2. Cephalic disproportion, which means the baby's skull is too big to pass through your pelvic outlet.
3. Severe fluctuations in the fetal heartbeat.

With each of these, you are likely to be in labor for a certain amount of time before your doctor decides on performing a ce-sarean. For instance, if the fetal heartbeat is irregular, you may be encouraged to lie on one side, or you may be given some oxygen before the decision is made to operate.

There are also reasons that demand a section for the baby's and your health. These are:

1. Active herpes.
2. A breech presentation of the baby.
3. Heart disease of the mother.
4. Diabetes of the mother.

Emergencies, which luckily are infrequent, would be:

1. Hemorrhaging of the mother.
2. Continuing very low fetal heart frequency.
3. Placenta Abrupta (premature rupture and expulsion of the placenta).

It usually does not take longer than about 4 to 5 minutes to deliver the baby by section. However, it does take at least 45 minutes to do the repair of the tissues. These days the cut is generally done horizontally (the bikini cut), which is not only aesthetically preferable but has the advantage of being in the toughest part of the uterine muscle, so that with a subsequent pregnancy there is a good chance of a vaginal delivery.

Even if you need to have a cesarean section, your Lamaze training will not be lost. Your ability to relax and the use of the breathing techniques during the immediate postpartum period will be of great benefit to you.

BEGINNING TO PUSH

If you are expecting your first baby, you will probably begin the second stage of labor, or expulsion of the baby, in the labor room. As I have emphasized before, *you must not push* until the doctor or midwife has given you permission to push. If you have forgotten how to push, let your husband supervise you. You will probably find that after one or two pushing contractions you will be able to follow the instructions that you have been given. Do not forget to take your pillows to the delivery room so that your head and back can be raised on the delivery table.

It is generally assumed that every woman will have an over-whelming urge to push once she is fully dilated. This is not always so. The majority of women do feel the strong expulsive urge; I have found that the urge to push varies in intensity from woman to woman. There are also some women who never feel any urge whatsoever. The latter may be due to the position or the rotation of the baby. Should you be one of those who does not feel the urge to push and your doctor tells you to push with the next contraction, don't argue, "But I don't feel like it yet." Accept your physician's orders at the time without questioning, and use the pushing technique with the next contraction regardless of whether you feel like it or not.

If you labor and deliver in the birthing room, your partner does not have to wear special sterile gown, cap and mask. In the delivery room, however, he will usually have to wear a cap, gown and mask. He will be told to stand next to your head and not to move from there unless he is asked to do so by your physician. You will be draped, and must remember to keep your hands firmly on the handles or stirrups. Remember, do not touch any of the sterile sheets. Before you start to push on the delivery table, the nurse will pour some disinfectant over your pubic area. This will feel icy cold, but it is actually quite a refreshing surprise!

BIRTHING ROOM AND BIRTHING CHAIR

Many hospitals offer birthing rooms these days. They are usually former labor rooms, which have been pleasantly furnished with drapes, often a carpet, a rocking chair for the woman to labor in, or for her partner to sit in. In short, a room with a homelike atmosphere. The bed is a labor-delivery bed, which means a comfortable bed that can be easily converted to become a comfortable delivery bed as well, where you do not have to lie flat in order to push your baby out. This means that a move to a different room, i.e., the delivery room, in the middle of pushing can be avoided.

Staying in the same place for the expulsion will conserve energy, and, of course, it will also give you a chance to deliver the baby in a sitting position, or a half-sitting position, on your side, or in any way you like and your doctor or midwife consider advisable at the time.

Some hospitals now also use a "birthing chair," which looks very much like a dentist's chair, which can be put into an upright position with your legs well supported. In this position, your doctor and your coach would be very close to you. You would form a little circle, working together, and the sense of working as a team can be greatly enhanced this way.

The birthing chair can also be tilted to place you on your back in a horizontal position, in case the doctor has to use forceps or any other maneuver that may be indicated to help your child safely into this world.

Your doctor will give you the command to push, once you are ready. Be sure to pant and blow whenever you are asked to stop pushing. This allows the doctor time to ease the baby along, to help deliver the head and shoulders, receiving the rest of the baby's body, which then slips out easily into his or her hands.

And so you have given birth to your baby! Your doctor or midwife will help your baby to take its first breath by gently sucking out the mucus from its mouth and nose. Then your baby will cry or make little sounds as it starts breathing on its own.

Babies do not come out looking washed and immaculate. Your baby will be wet and wrinkled. It will have patches of a whitish cream all over its body, which is the protective coating, or "vernix," which the baby had while growing in your uterus, and it will look bluish gray for a few seconds before it starts to cry and the color of its skin changes to pink. Black babies will look very light when born. Their pigmentation occurs gradually.

Your doctor will then put the baby on your abdomen. Remember, this is the sterile area, therefore an excellent place to put the baby while the umbilical cord is clamped and cut. But keep your hands under the drapes. You will have to wait just a little longer before you are allowed to hold your child.

Once the cord has been cut—which does not hurt either you or the baby—the nurse will wrap your baby in a warm blanket and put it into a bassinette, which is slightly tilted to help the baby expel more mucus and make breathing easier. The nurse will put a plastic identification band on the baby and on you. Your fingerprints may be taken and possibly the baby's footprints. A few drops of silver nitrate or antibiotic ointment may be put into the baby's eyes, or the baby may be given a penicillin shot instead.

A number of physicians and midwives adopt some of Dr. Leboyer's ideas these days. Also, many couples are asking that Leboyer's approach, i.e., "the baby is a person," be used. Lights are dimmed in the delivery room, except for a spotlight on the mother's pelvic floor. The baby stays for a longer period on the mother's abdomen so that she can touch it gently, rub its back and establish eye contact with her child.

A newborn baby can actually see at about one foot distance. Your baby will be looking at you, and you can establish the beginning of a long relationship by having eye contact, holding the baby and letting it get acquainted with you and your husband. It will feel different to the baby to be held by you, and your baby will soon recognize your special way of holding it, your smell and your voice.

If you are on an IV, a hormone will be given to you intravenously that will contract your uterus and help expel the placenta. If you are not on an IV, you may get an injection of this hormone. It will prevent excessive bleeding and start to reduce the uterus to its non-pregnant size. In the meantime, you may have another contraction. The doctor will feel your uterus and decide that it is time for you to "express" the placenta (our third stage of labor). Be sure to help the doctor with another good push to expel the placenta. The doctor will assist you by putting gentle pressure on your abdomen. It will take no more than two to three minutes to expel the placenta. Now your hard work is over.

If your doctor has performed an episiotomy, he/she will clean you up and perform "the repair" or stitching. While this is done, ask to hold your baby. Frequently you'll get to hold and talk to it while your doctor does the repair. Your husband will also hold and touch the baby and help you put the baby to your breast should you desire to nurse it right there and then.

Your partner's place is always next to you, so that he can talk to you, helping to raise your head and shoulders when you push, and perhaps reminding you to push either gently or a little more forcefully, as circumstances require. He can encourage you to remember how to push and perhaps give you the commands as each contraction occurs.

AFTER YOU'VE GIVEN BIRTH

For about two hours after you have given birth, a nurse will watch you closely. She will massage your abdomen from time to time to make sure that your uterus remains firm. Occasionally the nurse will show you how to massage your abdomen yourself.

Now you will be taken back to your own bed in your own room. You will probably feel fantastically elated! You may not be able to sleep much the first night after you've given birth.

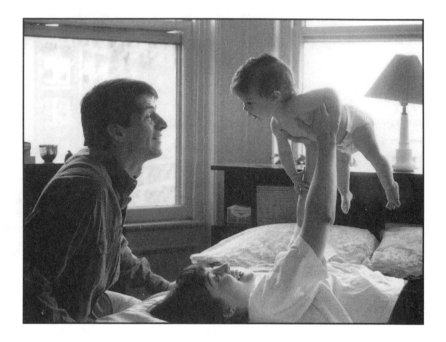

You'll be proud of your baby and of yourself, of your husband and of your ability to have functioned so well.

However, there is still some immediate work ahead of you. Do not forget to do your pelvic floor contractions; they will speed your recovery. Also you *will* experience some slight continued contractions, which are a good sign that your uterus is healing and contracting again to its original size. These contractions after childbirth will be more pronounced if this was your second, third or fourth delivery, since it becomes more difficult for the muscles to regain their original tone. You are also likely to feel them when you nurse your baby.

Please remember that these contractions occur for a very good reason: to get your uterus back to its usual size. They are a sign of a speedy recovery.

And so you have given birth to your baby. You have joined all the thousands of mothers and fathers who have trained themselves to give birth actively instead of passively, and you have prepared yourself diligently for the first step on the road to successful parenthood.

LABOR GUIDELINES FOR FATHERS OR COACHES

STAGE	MOTHER	FATHER OR COACH
FIRST STAGE OF LABOR		
1. *Early Labor* Effacement and dilation to 3–4 centimeters.	Great excitement and nervousness. Tendency to start breathing techniques too early. Possible breaking of bag of waters. Use first breathing technique, if necessary.	• Keep your partner company. Celebrate the beginning of the baby's birthday. • Encourage walking and normal activities if labor starts in daytime. • Encourage rest and sleep if it is nighttime. She will not miss out on her labor and sleep is the most important factor. • Light food intake for mother. • Rehearse Lamaze techniques once more. • Supervise first breathing technique if necessary. Time contractions.
2. *Active Labor* Dilation from about 3–8 centimeters.	Contractions are probably less than five minutes apart. Concentration is needed. Talking and joking will become less. First and second breathing techniques.	• Time contractions. Count aloud intervals of 15 seconds to make contraction seem to pass more quickly. • Watch for relaxation. Use technique of "touch" relaxation. Encourage change of positions. • Call doctor or midwife. Have Lamaze bag packed and ready. • Get car or taxi for trip to hospital. • Keep encouraging your partner, praising her efforts, and watching carefully for relaxation. • With second breathing technique, avoid too rapid breathing. Breathe with partner to establish rhythm. • Massage her abdomen, back or legs, if needed.

3. *Transition* Dilation from about 8–10 centimeters.	Panicky feeling of not being able to continue. Irritability, backache, slight bleeding. Possible shaking, nausea. Sometimes urge to push. Third breathing technique.	• Very concentrated help and encouragement. Remind her that she is almost at the end. Be firm and strong. • Breathe with your partner. Work with one and think of only one contraction at a time. Do not anticipate! This lasts about one hour. Remind her that she is working so hard for the baby. • Support her back, use counter pressure, use washcloth to refresh her face. Stroke legs gently and firmly to remove tension. Encourage. Praise.

SECOND STAGE

4. *Expulsion* From full dilation to the birth of the baby.	Urge to push, generally like an "inner force." Often a great relief.	• Remind her how to push. Sit on tailbone, at about 75° angle. Rest legs on bed. Hold on to knees, elbows out. • Give commands for pushing: Breathe in, exhale, inhale, exhale, inhale, exhale a little, keep mouth and throat open, push with residual air, exhale. Take another breath, let out half, push with residual air, do not close your throat. Continue until contraction is over. • Give your partner a running commentary when you see the head appear. She may be too busy to look. Encourage her to look in the mirror; she will probably push better when she sees the baby emerging. • Birth of baby. • Ecstasy. Joy. Love. Exhaustion. • Feeling of wonderful achievement and awe.

THIRD STAGE

5. Expulsion of the afterbirth or placenta.	Help pushing the placenta out. Doctor or midwife will assist with pressure on the abdomen.	• Encourage active pushing.

A MOTHER'S REPORT

BY PHYLIS FEINSTEIN

*A personal, moment-by-moment account
by a young woman, prepared with the
Lamaze method, of her first childbirth.*

The beginning of my labor was less than auspicious. My first indication that the baby would be born this year yet occurred Tuesday around 1:30 P.M. when my mucous plug came out. No contractions, no showing . . . nothing.

All afternoon I waited. About once every half hour I'd get a tiny tweak in my pelvic area, but it was so short and inconsequential that I'm not sure I didn't wish it into existence. I called Richard, my husband, a dozen times during the course of the day to tell him not to come home yet. However, I also informed him it could happen any minute.

For some reason every appliance in our house got serviced that Tuesday. And so the washing machine got its new grounding wire, the dryer a new catch, etc. I was busy answering the door all afternoon, feeling fine—if a little apprehensive. Checking my preparation for when labor would begin, I found a half bowl of Jell-O in the refrigerator (if I should get hungry during the earliest stages), a container of stew in the freezer (for

Richard to take to the hospital in a wide-mouthed thermos in case *he* got hungry), my luggage packed and my Lamaze goodie bag complete.

About the goodie bag: I had decided to make it particularly nice, figuring that at the time I would need it, any pleasantry would help. And so the bag itself was not an ordinary brown, dull grocery model. This was a slick-papered pink (prophetic) bag, the kind lazy gift-givers use instead of fancy wrapping paper on the outside of presents. Inside was a brand-new flowered washcloth—blue (unprophetic)—my favorite talc (we used practically the entire can), chapstick, some fancy lollipops, and the three-dollar-wonder of a clock I used to time my breathing exercises. The clock has a cracked face, no minute hand, but the niftiest second hand. I was confidently prepared . . . until 3:00 A.M. Wednesday morning, when the first real contraction lifted me out of a deep sleep. I bolted from my warm bed groaning, "My God, I've got back labor." Naturally this woke Richard, and for the next half hour all the careful planning, the long, intellectual discussions about not panicking were forgotten.

We were both in a maddening state of hysteria. I couldn't face having back labor.

Richard couldn't face that I was in labor and, after assuring me labor doesn't start this way, he said in his most condescending tone, "Obviously, you're constipated." Then he added, "Gee, I'm starving," and dove into the refrigerator.

Meanwhile I sat on a kitchen stool, effleuraging like mad, breathing properly and quietly swearing alternately at back labor and at my husband. I soon checked my contractions at five-minute intervals, when I mustered, "Richard, you'd better call the doctor."

Richard acquiesced. In his Cary Grant manner he began the conversation suavely, "Hello, Doctor. How are you?" (At 3:00 in the morning!) "Yes, this is Richard Feinstein. Phylis *thinks* she's in labor. Every five minutes. Clock them for another half hour and if they are steady call back? Call back anyway? O.K." By fifteen minutes later the contractions were coming every four minutes. We called our doctor again and were told to come nearer the hospital (we live half an hour away) and wait a bit at my cousin's, who lives only a block from the hospital. We forgot Richard's stew. But before we left he ate my Jell-O. And while I dressed he managed to brew some tea and pack some fruit for the trip. By this time I had hold of myself, and found the ride on the parkway uneventful. Richard concentrated on the road and I on my contractions. I cracked open the package of lollipops and lapped away when my mouth became dry. (First mistake: Don't buy sweet pops. The smaller, sourer ones are much better.) I had beside me two pillows I'd grabbed just in case the hospital was short-stocked. It proved to be good thinking!

We arrived at my cousin's at 4:00 A.M. The door was opened by two sleepy and excited relatives. Now my contractions were two minutes apart. Another call to the doctor and we were off to the hospital at last. We entered, Richard carrying my goodie bag and his box lunch and I clutching my pillows and sucking my too-sweet lollipop. We were quite a pair.

An o.b. nurse was sent down to accompany me to the maternity floor. In the elevator she looked me up and down, taking in my pillows and lollipop.

"Why those?" She pointed.

I said, "Pillows for back support. Pops for dry mouth."

Off the elevator she headed me toward a room I shared with

three other ladies. I readied for bed and, in between shallow breathing techniques, I asked a nurse to roll up my bed.

She did, muttering, "Everyone lies down for labor; you sit like a tailor sewing."

She left as Richard returned from signing me in. He dismantled the bag, placing the talc, washcloth, chapstick and lollies close by. The doctor arrived, followed by a blonde bulldozer of a nurse. She looked at Richard and said, "Better you wait in the solarium. Better still wait downstairs till it's over." In unison Richard and I said, "No, he's [I'm] going to stay." The nurse acquiesced and, looking offended, she left the room.

Richard timed my contractions; I rubbed my belly. Ten minutes later, Dr. H. broke my water. I was put on a movable table and taken to a private room, where Richard and I spent the entire labor.

We were finally settled and ready for action. For the first time I had a chance to evaluate what was happening inside me. I wasn't having true back labor because, Dr. H. assured me, the baby was not in a posterior position. The contractions began at the back, reached their peak about three inches below my navel and then spread in both directions toward my hips as they subsided. I was breathing as directed in the second stage of the first part of labor (dilation)—cleansing breath, slow breath, acceleration as the contraction built and then regaining a slow pace as it lessened. The doctor examined me at 5:30 and told us what was going on. The only time he asked me if I wanted any medication was about 4:30 A.M. He said it to reassure me, I guess. But he never offered it again. Even when the going got tough during the last stage of transition. After the birth, I asked why he never again mentioned it. His answer: "Who needed it?"

By 8:00 I was 9½ centimeters and fagged out. I wanted to push, but Dr. H. said not yet. I wanted to push *very* badly. I lost my breathing, grabbed for Richard's and Dr. H.'s hands, blew out all my good oxygen and squeezed their hands. "It's time," I moaned. Dr. H's examination showed I was wrong. The cervix had just a little left to dilate, enough to make a difference between pushing uselessly and productive expulsion. Meanwhile Richard got me on the road to breathing properly by forcing me to listen to him do it. Thirty minutes later came the word—*push!* I got into position (after Richard reminded me to *get* into position) and I pushed. Erroneously I thought three good pushes and out would come baby. Ha!

The hardest part, for me, was the expulsion. It hurt and I was tired. "No more pushing," I groaned, just as the doctor said, "Come here, Richard—here comes your baby's head and the hair's black." Rich rushed around the bed. Then I grinned and said, "Who's tired?" I wanted to push more than anything else in the world.

They took us to the delivery room. Dr. H. administered a local for the episiotomy. What seemed like five pushes—good ones—and then minutes later the doctor lifted up the biggest, most beautiful girl baby I've ever seen: 8 pounds, 2 ounces, 21 inches of Lamaze testimonial.

I don't know words to describe it.

A FATHER'S REPORT

BY PATRICK CASEY

*The role of the partner is crucial throughout labor and
delivery; here is one man's report of his experience.*

The birth of our first child had been an unpleasant experience.
My wife had no real idea of what to expect when those first
contractions came four years ago. She was surprised, frightened
and extremely uncomfortable. Neither of us had any notion
that childbirth could be such a harrowing ordeal. After a few
moments of desperate handholding I was asked to leave the
hospital room; she was heavily medicated and, at the end of
several hours of anxiety and confusion, I was informed that our
first son had arrived. Happily, he was a fine, healthy baby, but
the experience was so distressing that for a long time Marilyn
would not consider going through the whole thing again.

Eventually we did decide to have another child. About the
same time Marilyn became pregnant again a friend told us
about a marvelous technique of childbirth called the Lamaze
method. A clear idea of what happens physically during labor
and delivery, a few exercises to prepare the body, a system of
breathing to alleviate discomfort during contractions *and* a

supporting role for the husband—it sounded practical, worth investigating. Certainly we wanted to do something to avoid another traumatic experience, so we went to an obstetrician who encouraged the Lamaze method and enrolled in the six-lesson course.

Those weekly sessions were really quite marvelous. Not only did they lift the traditional veil of mystery about childbirth by simply explaining what was going to happen and how to prepare for it, but they helped eliminate any nervous apprehension about the whole event. By creating a warm atmosphere of rational discussion, and by giving us specific exercises and techniques to practice together, the classes gradually dispelled our anxieties. We aired our questions with the other four couples in the class; we worked together at home. The whole thing became a happy collaboration, something we were preparing for as husband and wife.

The first contractions came at about 3:00 A.M. a few days after the anticipated date of delivery. Marilyn woke me at 3:30, announcing that she had been having what "could be real contractions" for half an hour. By 4:00 A.M. I was calling Dr. A. to report regular mild contractions about five minutes apart. We knew that a second baby usually comes faster than the first, but we were surprised to hear him tell us to get down to the hospital as quickly as we could. Marilyn's suitcase and the little Lamaze bag had both been carefully packed weeks before. Without further delay we hopped in a cab.

Marilyn's water hadn't broken yet—the first thing that happened when Jonathan was born—but as we sped toward the hospital her contractions continued to be definite and regular. I suggested that she begin the first breathing technique, but she refused, reminding me that we had been taught to wait until it was absolutely necessary. At 4:30 we pulled up to the night entrance of the hospital.

We had registered and left a deposit with the hospital a month before, so we went straight up to the fourth-floor delivery area where Dr. A. was already waiting. In a wonderfully encouraging manner he took Marilyn into the labor room to be dressed and examined while I changed into regulation sterile-white shirt and pants next door. About ten minutes later I joined Marilyn in the labor room, where one pillow was under her head and another under her knees. She told me that she was already 5 centimeters dilated and would allegedly have the baby within the hour. It was now 4:45 A.M. We were both terribly excited as she began doing the accelerated breathing. I made myself useful by powdering her abdomen and giving her a lollipop to suck on between contractions. Marilyn laughed at my hospital get-up. She thought it would be a girl. I was noncommittal.

A friendly nurse bustled in and out, while a resident technician took a sample of blood. The contractions had been mild and relatively close together, but now were getting slightly stronger and more difficult to control. It was exactly like our practice at home: Marilyn breathed and concentrated on a spot across the little room, while I called off fifteen-second intervals of the contraction.

At 5:10 things quickened; Marilyn began having really strong contractions. Immediately we shifted into the rapid breathing and blowing method of breathing. The doctor came in, made a quick examination and called for the nurse; we were going into the delivery room! I grabbed two pillows and tried to keep up with the rolling table, while fitting on my cap and face mask. The nurse laughed at me as I trotted along, dropping a pillow every three feet, but dauntlessly following everyone into the delivery room where Marilyn was already being transferred to the table. Now the contractions were quite intense and she really had to hold back the urge to push and force herself to concentrate on breathing.

The atmosphere in the delivery room was something like a congenial clubhouse. I was introduced to the anesthesiologist ("He's here just in case we need any medication.") and to the two nurses who were performing little chores about the room with towels and instruments. The baby's head was about to show, the doctor told us, and with the next contraction he would break the membranes and Marilyn could at last begin to push. I mopped her brow, which really wasn't at all necessary, and tried to keep busy arranging the pillows beneath her head.

"Ready," Dr. A. said quietly, as Marilyn took her two deep breaths, took a third breath, let out a little air, and pushed with the remaining breath, while I counted to eight. A fierce growl-like noise filled the room as she bared her teeth, straining down and out, gripping the metal bars of the table. I think she must have been oblivious to everything else in the room, so powerful was her concentration and determination. A gush of water shot across the room.

"Good!" the doctor said, ". . . and again . . ."

The incredible noise she made! And the strength of her face. It was like watching some legendary hero perform a Herculean triumph, toppling a temple, overthrowing a false god, defeating an enemy.

"Very good! Come and look—you can see the baby's hair."

I rushed to peer over the doctor's shoulder. There was the top of the baby's head, plastered with what looked then like dark hair.

Marilyn gave a faint smile and prepared to push again. At this point the doctor gave Marilyn an injection of local anesthetic and made an incision, painlessly, to enlarge the opening. One last push and I saw the head come completely out. Dr. A. worked his hand under the shoulder and in a second the whole child slid easily into the world.

"It's a boy!" the anesthesiologist said, first to notice from his vantage point at Marilyn's head. "The time is 5:37."

It was indeed a boy, looking quite wrinkled and angry. Being a naturally anxious sort, I was relieved to note that he had only one head, two arms, two legs, etc. His skin had a bluish tinge, as he hung from the doctor's grip, and his little body was tense. The umbilical cord ran from his navel to the placenta, which had not yet been expelled. The cord was clamped and cut, while I fretted about his lifeless appearance. The doctor then gave him a slap on the soles of his feet. (Apparently, spanking the bottom is only for the movies.) There was a gurgle deep in the baby's throat, in another second a faint cry, and then a series of lusty yells and wails. He was really alive—very much so!

Dr. A. ordered another short push to expel the placenta, and in no time at all he had stitched up the episiotomy. In the meantime, we could not take our eyes off little Peter Nicholas (for that was to be his name), who was getting pinker and pinker in the glass box he had been placed in next to the delivery table. We could see now that what I had thought was dark hair was really wet red hair, exactly the same shade as his mother's and brother's.

Then we were left quite alone. The anesthesiologist packed up his tanks and left. The nurses were in and out, and the doctor went off to see about another woman who had arrived in labor.

It was the proudest, happiest moment of our lives. Here was our new son, after only two hours of mild labor and absolutely no medication whatsoever, not even an aspirin! The difference between this and our first childbirth was miraculous. Marilyn had used the Lamaze method to perfection. The method had given us calmness with which we both approached the event, confidence with which we were able to cope with each succeeding stage, joy in doing all this together and this ultimate, happy reward.

ABOUT THE AUTHOR

ELISABETH BING was born in Berlin, Germany, of a distinguished scientific family. She was trained as a physical therapist in London, England, and came to New York in 1949. She worked under Dr. Alan Guttmacher in the Childbirth Education Program at the Mt. Sinai Hospital from 1952 until 1960. Elisabeth Bing became one of the co-founders of the American Society for Psychoprophylaxis in Obstetrics, Inc. in 1960. Since then she has been a member of the department of obstetrics and gynecology of the N.Y. Medical College. Elisabeth Bing has trained thousands of expectant parents in her own private classes. She has traveled widely all over the U.S. and Europe, giving workshops, lecturing and holding seminars in many colleges, hospitals and communities. She is the author of six books on childbirth education.

For information about Lamaze-oriented doctors, midwives, and childbirth instructors in your area, you may contact:

The American Society for Psychoprophylaxis in Obstetrics (ASPO/LAMAZE)
1101 Connecticut Ave., NW
Suite 700
Washington, DC 20036
(800) 368-4404 or (202) 857-1128

ASPO also provides workshops, teacher training, and parent-division activities.